Quick Fix
Acupressure Method
Pain-Free in Minutes

Dr. Constance Santego

Maximillian Enterprises
Kelowna, BC

Quick Fix Acupressure Method

Copyright © 2025 by Dr. Constance Santego.

Copy Editor & Interior Design: Constance Santego
Book Layout: ©2017 BookDesignTemplates.com

Ordering Information:
Quantity sales. Special discounts are available on quantity purchases by corporations, associations, and others. For details, contact the "Special Sales Department" at the address above.

Trade Paperback 978-1-990062-79-7
Ebook ISBN 978-1-990062-80-3
Created and published In Canada. Printed and bound in the United States of America

First Edition
Published by Maximillian Enterprises
Kelowna, BC
Canada
www.constancesantego.ca

Dedication

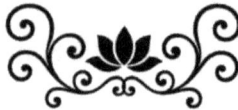

To the healers who came before me, for building the foundation, and to my students, clients, and readers, who continue to remind me why this work matters. May you always remember: your body was designed to heal.

"The natural healing force within each of us is the greatest force in getting well."
—Hippocrates

ALSO BY DR. CONSTANCE SANTEGO

NOVELS

Illegitimate Grace
Ashcroft Hollow

Okanagan Trilogy:
Beneath the Vineyards
Under the Okanagan Sun
Guardian of the Lake

The Nine Spiritual Gifts Series:
Journey of a Soul – (Vol 1 Michael)
Language of a Soul – (Vol 2 Gabriel)
Prophecy of a Soul – (Vol 3 Bath Kol)
Healing of a Soul – (Vol 4 Raphael)
Miracles of a Soul – (Vol 5 Hamied)
Knowledge of a Soul – (Vol 6 Raziel)
Wisdom of a Soul – (Vol 7 Uriel)
Faith of a Soul – (Vol 8 Pistis Sophia)

NONFICTION
The Intuitive Life, The Gift Of Prophecy, Third Edition
Fairy Tales, Dreams And Reality... Where Are You On Your Path?
Second Edition
Your Persona... The Mask You Wear
Archangel Michael's Soul Retrieval Guide
Tesla And The Future Of Energy Medicine
Beyond Tesla: Advancing The Science Of Energy Healing
Tesla's Code: Mastering Energy, Frequency, And Creative Power
Beyond The Mind: Harnessing The Power Of Astral Projection For
Creative Awakening
Bend, Don't Break: Finding Your Way Back To Abundance
Ring Therapy: A Guide To Healing And Balance
Ring Therapy Pocket Guide
Floraopathy™: The Art And Science Of Vibrational Healing With
Essential Oils
Dear Older Me: A Memoir... *Of Sorts*
It's Just Like Poker: A Spiritual Guide To Playing The
Cards Life Deals You
Signs And Meanings: What The Feet Reveal About Health, Stress,
and the Body's Story
Auricions: Unlocking Subconscious Healing Through Quantum
Medicine |

Type 3 Diabetes: The Hidden Link Between Blood Sugar, Brain
Health, And Healing Naturally

REIKI WISDOM, SERIES:
Angelic Lifestyle, a Vibrant Lifestyle
Angelic Lifestyle 42-Day Energy Cleanse
Reiki and the Power of The Joint Points: Unlocking Energy Pathways
for Healing
Reiki and Karmic Healing: Releasing Patterns From Past Reiki and
the Five Elements
Secrets of a Healer, Magic Of Reiki
The Reiki Master's Manual

SECRETS OF A HEALER, SERIES:
Magic Of Aromatherapy (Vol I)
Magic Of Reflexology (Vol II)
Magic Of The Gifts (Vol III)
Magic Of Muscle Testing (Vol IV)
Magic Of Iridology (Vol V)
Magic Of Massage (Vol VI)
Magic Of Hypnotherapy (Vol VII)
Magic Of Reiki (Vol VIII)
Magic Of Advanced Aromatherapy (Vol IX)
Magic Of Esthetics (Vol X)
The Reiki Master's Manual (Vol XI)

ADULT COLORING JOURNALS
SERIES-ZEN COLORING:
Quantum Energy and Mindful Living Journal (Vol 1)
Reiki Energy Journal (Vol 2)
Nine Spiritual Gifts Journal (Vol 3)
I Forgive Journal (Vol 4)

FOR CHILDREN
I am Big Tonight. I Don't Need the Light

COOKBOOK
My Favorite Recipes, with a Hint of Giggle

BUISNESS
How To Use ChatGPT For Authors: From Idea to Published Book
Scaling Beyond 6 Figures: Strategies for Health & Wellness
Professionals
The Academypreneur's Playbook: Turn Knowledge Into A
Revenue-Generating School

Contents

Preface

A Lineage of Healing at Our Fingertips

Every healing method we use today has roots—threads of wisdom passed down through practitioners who observed, experimented, and refined techniques over generations. *The Quick Fix Pain Relief Method* is not something created in isolation; it is part of a long lineage of innovators who believed in the body's innate ability to heal when given the right stimulus.

The story begins with **D.D. Palmer**, who in 1895 introduced chiropractic care and the concept of *Innate Intelligence*. Palmer taught that the body has a natural, self-healing force and that spinal adjustments could remove interference to this flow. His revolutionary idea set the stage for countless integrative therapies.

In the **1930s**, **Dr. Terrence Bennett** discovered neurovascular reflex points—specific spots on the body where light touch could stimulate circulation and restore function. Around the same time, **Dr. De Jarnette** advanced the Sacro-Occipital Technique, focusing on the vital relationship between the pelvis, cranium, and nervous system. Both men added depth and dimension to Palmer's foundation, blending structural and energetic perspectives.

By the **1960s**, **Dr. George Goodheart** built upon these discoveries to create *Applied Kinesiology*, combining muscle testing with reflex points, chiropractic, nutrition, and Traditional Chinese Medicine. Goodheart's system opened the door to understanding how structural, chemical, and emotional imbalances reveal themselves through the body.

Dr. John Thie, one of Goodheart's students, took these complex ideas and translated them for the everyday person. In the **1970s**, he published *Touch for Health*, a breakthrough self-care guide that empowered ordinary people to balance their energy, reduce pain, and improve well-being without needing a professional degree.

It is upon this remarkable foundation that the **Quick Fix Method** rests. My contribution has been to streamline these principles into a **fast, accessible sequence** that anyone can use—without advanced training, expensive equipment, or complicated protocols. By focusing on **neuro-lymphatic points** and simple breathwork, Quick Fix offers relief in moments while honoring the wisdom of those who came before.

This book is both a continuation and a simplification of that lineage—a way to place healing literally back into your own hands.

What began as a journey through my own studies and healing experiences has grown into a method I am honored to share with you. Quick Fix is more than a technique—it is a reminder that your body is wise, resilient, and ready to heal.

In faith and healing,
Dr. Constance Santego

Note to Reader

The Quick Fix Method is not meant to replace modern medicine. Your doctor still plays an essential role in your health and well-being. If I were to break my leg, I would absolutely rely on a doctor, along with the nurses and staff in the hospital, to set the bone and care for me properly.

What this book offers is something different—something complementary. In Eastern medicine, there is a deep belief that we each play an active role in maintaining our own health, rather than leaving it entirely to doctors to repair us after illness or injury has taken hold. Eastern approaches focus on balance: caring for body, mind, and spirit; reducing stress; nurturing vital energy; and being mindful of what we allow into both our bodies and our thoughts.

The Quick Fix Method uses acupressure on neuro-lymphatic points as a practical tool to support this balance. It is a simple technique that allows you to connect with your body, listen to its messages, and respond with honesty and intention. By developing sensitivity to your body's feedback, you begin to create a path toward greater health and harmony—for your body, your mind, and your soul.

Shift happens...Create magic!

Learning Outcome

When you have completed this book and practiced the Quick Fix techniques, you will:

- Understand the basics of **acupressure and neuro-lymphatic points**, and how they influence the body's natural energy flow.
- Learn a **simple step-by-step Quick Fix sequence** to reduce pain in minutes and restore balance.
- Gain confidence in using your **hands, breath, and intention** as healing tools.
- Recognize the **five types of pain**—physical, emotional, energetic, stress-related, and referred—and how to approach each with acupressure.
- Discover how the **Five Element Theory** supports balance of body, mind, and spirit.
- Explore ways to combine Quick Fix with other self-care practices, including **aromatherapy, visualization, and breathwork**.
- Build a **personal practice** that can be used daily—for immediate relief, long-term well-being, and a deeper connection to your body's wisdom.

Quick Fix
Acupressure Method

Pain-Free in Minutes

Dr. Constance Santego

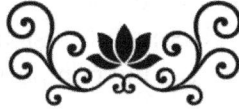

Why We Need a Quick Fix for Pain

Pain has a way of stopping life in its tracks. Whether it's the sudden grip of a headache, the ache of tight shoulders after a stressful day, or the lingering throb of an old injury, pain steals our focus, our energy, and sometimes even our joy. For many, the immediate solution is to reach for a pill, push through it, or simply accept discomfort as part of daily life.

But what if relief didn't have to mean medication, side effects, or waiting for the pain to "go away on its own"? What if there were a simple, natural method you could use—right in the moment—to ease your discomfort and restore balance in just minutes?

That is why the Quick Fix Method exists.

We live in a world that moves fast. Most people don't have the time, resources, or energy to book endless appointments or commit to complicated healing systems. We need something practical—something we can use *anytime, anywhere*—whether in the middle of a workday, on a long commute, or at home when pain suddenly strikes. Quick Fix is designed for exactly that purpose: to empower you with a straightforward sequence of acupressure points that can be applied in just minutes, bringing immediate relief while also supporting the deeper balance of your body's energy.

This approach does not replace medical care, but it gives you back a sense of control. It is a reminder that your body carries within it remarkable wisdom and the ability to heal. By learning how to tap into that wisdom, you no longer have to feel powerless in the face of discomfort. Instead, you can respond to pain with confidence, clarity, and compassion for yourself.

Quick Fix is more than a technique—it is a philosophy. It says that relief should be accessible, that healing should be simple, and that every person deserves to feel at home in their own body.

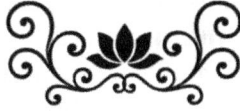

My Journey with Acupressure & Healing

In 1997, I began working at a Natural Health Clinic. At first, I was hired to practice the Emotional Polarity Technique, but before long, the clinic started training me in other modalities. My very first course was in **Iridology**. I remember thinking, *"Wonderful—I can now see what's happening inside the body. But how do I actually help fix it?"* That question stayed with me.

Soon, I added **massage** and then **Touch for Health** kinesiology to my training. Within a year, I had also become a **Reiki practitioner** and felt ready to step out on my own.

During those early years, I noticed one thing again and again: **pain was the common denominator.** Nearly every client who came through my door was struggling with some form of pain. And truthfully, I was too.

Before entering natural health, I owned an **industrial sewing business**—just as my mother had before me. But after having two children, my back began to give out. Something as simple as bending down to pick up a pencil could leave me collapsed on the floor in agony, unable to move for days. The chiropractor could realign my spine, but the relief never lasted. Eventually, I was forced to sell the business I had worked so hard to build. That painful ending became the doorway to an entirely new career.

The real turning point came when I discovered the **neuro-lymphatic massage technique**. For the first time, I experienced not just temporary relief, but lasting stability. Chiropractic adjustments could align me—but rubbing the neuro-lymphatic points **kept me aligned**. It was a revelation.

As I practiced with clients, I began adapting the Touch for Health method into something more focused and practical. I started asking clients to identify their pain on a **scale from 1 to 10** (with 10 being severe). Then I would guide them through a full sequence of neuro-lymphatic point stimulation, encouraging them to copy my movements. After a brief "shimmy" to reset the body, we would reassess. Almost every time, their pain had **dropped significantly**. Repeating the sequence a second time often reduced the pain to **zero**.

One client was so impressed that he asked to see the chart I was using. A few days later, he returned with a version of his own design—a gift that later inspired the chart I use to this very day.

Over time, I discovered something even more profound: this method wasn't only working on **physical pain**. It also eased **emotional pain**—releasing grief, calming anxiety, and softening the weight of stress. It was then that I realized I had found the tool I had been searching for all along: a simple, repeatable sequence that empowers people to heal themselves.

That discovery became the foundation for what I now call the **Quick Fix Method**—the system you are about to learn in this book.

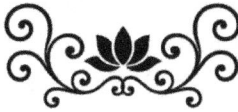

How to Use This Book

This book is designed to be **practical, simple, and ready to use**—whether you want to learn the philosophy behind the Quick Fix Method or you just need immediate relief right now.

You don't have to read it cover to cover to benefit. Think of it as both a **guidebook** and a **toolbox**:

- **If you're curious about the "why" behind pain and healing** → start with **Part I: Understanding Pain and Healing**, where you'll learn how pain works, the role of energy, and why acupressure is so effective.
- **If you're ready to start applying Quick Fix right away** → go directly to **Part II: The Quick Fix Method**, where you'll find step-by-step instructions and the Quick Fix Chart to guide you through the sequence.
- **If you want to create lasting habits** → explore **Part III: Living Pain-Free**, which shows you how to integrate Quick Fix into daily life and combine it with other holistic tools for long-term well-being.
- **When you just need a quick answer** → flip to the **Appendices**, where you'll find clear charts, quick-reference sequences, and blank journal pages to track your progress.

The methods you'll discover here are safe, natural, and adaptable. The more you practice, the more quickly your body will respond. Each time you use Quick Fix, you'll strengthen your awareness of your body's signals and your confidence in responding to them.

Keep this book close—by your bedside, in your bag, or on your desk—so that whenever pain interrupts your day, you have an immediate way to restore balance, energy, and relief.

Part I: Understanding Pain and Healing

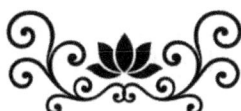

What Pain Really Means

Pain is more than just an unpleasant sensation—it is your body's way of communicating. Like a warning light on the dashboard of a car, pain signals that something needs attention. Too often, we treat pain as the enemy to be silenced rather than as a message to be understood.

PAIN AS A MESSENGER

At its core, pain is a **protective mechanism**. It alerts us to injury, imbalance, or stress before greater harm occurs. For example:

- A sudden sharp pain may stop you from moving in a way that would cause further damage.
- A dull, ongoing ache may signal that you are overusing a muscle or holding stress in your body.
- Emotional pain may indicate unresolved tension that is affecting both your mind and physical health.

When we ignore or suppress pain without listening to its source, we miss the opportunity to understand what our body is truly asking for.

THE MANY FACES OF PAIN

Pain is not one-size-fits-all. It can be:

- **Physical:** stemming from injury, posture, or strain.
- **Emotional:** rooted in stress, grief, or unresolved trauma.
- **Energetic:** caused by blockages in the flow of chi (life energy).
- **Stress-induced:** triggered by lifestyle, fatigue, or overwhelm.
- **Referred:** where the pain shows up in one place but originates elsewhere in the body.

Recognizing these layers of pain is the first step in knowing how to respond.

FROM SYMPTOM TO SIGNAL

Rather than asking *"How do I make the pain stop?"* the deeper question is:
"What is my body trying to tell me?"

By shifting your perspective, pain transforms from something to be feared into a guide—a signal pointing you toward balance, healing, and awareness.

THE ROLE OF QUICK FIX

The Quick Fix Method does not erase the importance of professional medical care when it's needed. Instead, it provides a **fast, supportive way to respond to pain as it arises**, relieving immediate discomfort while helping you uncover the underlying imbalances.

In this way, Quick Fix works in harmony with your body, empowering you to participate actively in your own healing.

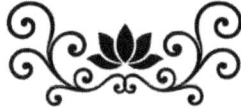

Acute vs. Chronic Pain

Not all pain is the same. Some forms of pain appear suddenly, demand attention, and then fade as the body recovers. Others linger for weeks, months, or even years, becoming woven into daily life. Understanding the difference between **acute** and **chronic** pain is essential—not only for proper care, but also for knowing how to apply the Quick Fix Method effectively.

ACUTE PAIN: THE BODY'S ALARM SYSTEM

Acute pain is short-term, usually lasting a few days to a few weeks. It often results from:

- An injury (like a sprain, cut, or burn)
- Overuse or strain (lifting something too heavy)
- Illness or infection
- Surgery or medical procedure

This type of pain acts as an **alarm bell**—loud, urgent, and protective. It tells you: *"Stop what you're doing and pay attention."* Once the underlying cause heals, the pain typically subsides.

Quick Fix can be very useful in acute situations. For example, applying acupressure to neuro-lymphatic points may reduce the intensity of muscle tension or discomfort, making it easier for your body to rest and heal. But remember: acute pain that is severe, sudden, or unexplained always deserves professional medical evaluation.

CHRONIC PAIN: WHEN THE ALARM KEEPS RINGING

Chronic pain lasts for months or even years. It may start with an injury that never fully healed, or it may arise without a clear cause. Examples include:

- Back pain that persists for years
- Migraines or frequent headaches
- Fibromyalgia and similar conditions
- Pain associated with stress, trauma, or emotional patterns

Chronic pain is more complex. Over time, the nervous system can become *hypersensitive*, amplifying pain signals even after the original injury has resolved. Emotional stress and energy blockages may also feed the cycle, keeping the body in a state of tension.

Here, Quick Fix becomes more than just a tool for immediate relief—it becomes part of a **daily practice of balance and release**. Each time you use the sequence, you interrupt the pain cycle, calm the nervous system, and remind your body how to reset.

WHY THE DISTINCTION MATTERS

- **Acute pain** tells you what needs care *right now*.
- **Chronic pain** tells you that your body has been asking for care for a long time.

Both deserve attention, but the approach differs. Acute pain calls for rest, protection, and support. Chronic pain calls for consistent, gentle interventions that address not only the physical body, but also the emotional, energetic, and stress-related roots.

QUICK FIX PERSPECTIVE

Quick Fix does not claim to cure either acute or chronic conditions. Instead, it offers a **bridge**: a way to quiet the noise of pain so you can listen more clearly to what your body needs. Whether you are soothing a sudden tension headache or softening the daily ache of tight shoulders, the Quick Fix Method gives you tools to take back a measure of control—one breath, one point, one moment at a time.

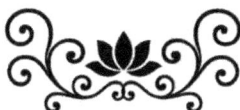

The Body's Messages: Listening to Symptoms

Your body is always speaking. Every ache, every spasm, every wave of fatigue is a message—yet in our busy lives, we often ignore these signals until they grow too loud to be dismissed. Pain is not random; it is your body's way of asking for attention, balance, and care.

SYMPTOMS AS SIGNALS

Think of your body as an intelligent messenger system. Symptoms are like **warning lights on a dashboard**—not the problem itself, but an indication that something beneath the surface requires attention.

For example:

- A tension headache may be your body's way of saying you're dehydrated, stressed, or pushing too hard.
- Shoulder pain may reflect more than muscle strain—it can reveal emotional burdens, unspoken worries, or energetic blocks.
- Digestive discomfort may point to diet, but also to the way you "process" experiences in your life.

When we treat only the surface symptom—masking the pain with medication or ignoring it altogether—we turn off the light without fixing what caused it to come on.

THE LANGUAGE OF PAIN

Each type of pain has its own "dialect":

- **Sharp, sudden pain**: an immediate warning—"Stop, pay attention now."
- **Dull, achy pain**: a reminder of something unresolved— "You've been holding on too long."
- **Recurring pain**: a repetitive message—"You haven't listened yet, so I'll keep asking."

By slowing down and observing the qualities of your pain, you begin to understand its meaning.

FROM RESISTANCE TO CURIOSITY

Most of us have been conditioned to fight pain, to see it as an enemy. But what if instead of resisting, you asked:

- *What is this sensation trying to tell me?*
- *Where in my life am I carrying stress or tension?*
- *What support is my body asking for right now?*

This shift—from frustration to curiosity—changes everything. Suddenly, pain is no longer just something to endure, but a teacher guiding you toward balance.

QUICK FIX AS A LISTENING TOOL

The Quick Fix Method is more than a technique for relief—it's a way of learning your body's language. Each time you press a neuro-lymphatic point, breathe, and reassess your pain level, you are entering into a **dialogue with your body**. The practice itself says: *I hear you. I'm responding.*

When you honor your symptoms as messages rather than nuisances, you unlock the wisdom behind them. Pain is not here to punish you—it is here to point the way back to balance.

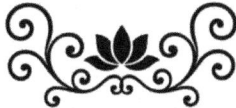

When Pain Is Not Muscular

Not all pain comes from muscles. While tension, strain, and injury are common causes, sometimes the source of discomfort lies deeper—or elsewhere altogether. Understanding when pain is not muscular helps you know how to respond, when to use Quick Fix, and when to seek other support.

PAIN THAT COMES FROM WITHIN

Some pain originates in the body's internal systems rather than the muscles or joints. For example:

- **Digestive issues** may cause abdominal cramping or back discomfort.

- **Kidney problems** can create pain in the lower back or sides.
- **Lung or heart conditions** may produce pain felt in the shoulders, chest, or even the arms.

These types of pain may feel muscular on the surface but actually reflect something happening in the organs.

REFERRED PAIN

Referred pain happens when discomfort is felt in one part of the body but originates elsewhere. For example:

- Pain in the left arm or jaw during a heart attack.
- Shoulder pain that actually stems from gallbladder stress.
- Sciatic pain down the leg is caused by a spinal nerve root compression.

Referred pain is a reminder that the body is interconnected—nerves, organs, muscles, and energy systems all communicate and influence one another.

EMOTIONAL AND ENERGETIC PAIN

Pain does not always have a purely physical cause. Emotional trauma, unresolved grief, or ongoing stress can manifest as tight muscles, headaches, or fatigue. Energetic imbalances—blockages in the body's natural flow of chi—can also produce sensations of heaviness, pressure, or discomfort.

This is why people sometimes say, *"I carry stress in my shoulders"* or *"My stomach is in knots."* The body records what the mind and emotions experience.

WHEN TO SEEK MEDICAL CARE

It's important to recognize when pain requires medical evaluation. Warning signs include:

- Sudden, severe, or unexplained pain.
- Pain accompanied by shortness of breath, dizziness, or chest pressure.
- Persistent pain that does not improve or worsens over time.
- Pain linked with fever, unexplained weight loss, or other concerning symptoms.

Quick Fix is a supportive tool, but it is not a replacement for professional diagnosis or treatment.

THE QUICK FIX ROLE

Even when pain is not muscular, Quick Fix can still help. By stimulating neuro-lymphatic points, you can:

- Reduce tension in the surrounding muscles.
- Support circulation and energy flow.
- Calm the nervous system, reducing the stress response.

While it may not cure the root cause of non-muscular pain, Quick Fix can make you more comfortable, more resilient, and better prepared to address the underlying issue.

Pain is a messenger, and sometimes the message points beyond muscles. By learning to distinguish the source, you gain clarity on when to use Quick Fix, when to explore deeper layers of healing, and when to seek medical care.

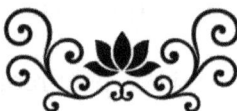

The Science Behind Acupressure

NEURO-LYMPHATIC POINTS EXPLAINED

To understand why the Quick Fix Method works, we need to explore the fascinating relationship between the body's nervous system, lymphatic system, and energy flow. The specific points used in Quick Fix are known as **neuro-lymphatic reflex points**—discovered in the early 1900s by Dr. Frank Chapman and later integrated into chiropractic, kinesiology, and energy medicine practices.

WHAT ARE NEURO-LYMPHATIC POINTS?

Neuro-lymphatic points are small, sensitive spots located mainly on the chest, ribs, abdomen, back, and legs. When massaged or stimulated, these points:

- Increase **lymphatic drainage**, helping clear toxins and waste products from tissues.
- Improve **circulation** of both blood and lymph.
- Activate the **autonomic nervous system**, helping muscles and organs return to balance.
- Relieve tension and restore energy flow along the body's meridian pathways.

In other words, they act like "reset buttons" for the body—removing blockages and improving communication between systems.

HOW THEY WERE DISCOVERED

- **Dr. Frank Chapman (1930s)** first mapped these reflex points and noticed that tender nodules under the skin corresponded to organ stress or imbalance. Gentle massage of these points improved function.
- **Dr. Terrence Bennett** expanded this work by identifying **neurovascular points** (on the head) that increased blood flow when touched.
- Later, **Dr. George Goodheart** (Applied Kinesiology) and **Dr. John Thie** (*Touch for Health*) integrated Chapman's neuro-lymphatic points into simple muscle-balancing protocols—making them accessible to practitioners and eventually the public.

HOW NEURO-LYMPHATIC POINTS RELIEVE PAIN

When a muscle is tight, weak, or overloaded, lymph flow often stagnates, and the surrounding tissue becomes tender. By massaging the related neuro-lymphatic point:

- Blockages in the lymphatic system are released.
- The nervous system calms, reducing pain signals.
- Muscles regain strength and flexibility.
- The body's natural healing processes are supported.

This is why pressing or massaging certain points can bring almost immediate relief—sometimes in just a few breaths.

WHY QUICK FIX USES THEM

The Quick Fix Method focuses on a handful of key neuro-lymphatic points because:

1. They can be reached easily without advanced training.
2. They produce **fast, noticeable results** when used in sequence.

3. They work on multiple levels—physical, energetic, and emotional.

By combining these points into one simple routine, you have a practical way to access the body's built-in healing system in minutes.

A BRIDGE BETWEEN SCIENCE AND ENERGY

While neuro-lymphatic points are well-documented in chiropractic and kinesiology, their effects also resonate with Traditional Chinese Medicine. The concept of **moving lymph and blood** mirrors the idea of restoring **chi (life force energy)**. Modern research on acupressure, lymphatic massage, and nervous system regulation is beginning to validate what healers have known for centuries: when flow is restored, pain diminishes and balance returns.

MERIDIANS, ENERGY FLOW, AND BALANCE

Beyond their physical effects on the lymph and nervous system, neuro-lymphatic points also connect to the body's **energy pathways**, called **meridians** in Traditional Chinese Medicine (TCM).

Meridians are invisible channels through which **chi** (life force energy) flows. Each meridian corresponds to a specific organ or system and influences both physical function and emotional states. For example:

- The **Stomach Meridian** is linked not only to digestion but also to worry and overthinking.
- The **Lung Meridian** influences breathing as well as feelings of grief or letting go.
- The **Liver Meridian** supports detoxification and is often tied to feelings of frustration or anger.

When chi flows smoothly through the meridians, the body feels energized, balanced, and resilient. When the flow is blocked or sluggish, pain, fatigue, or emotional tension may appear.

HOW ACUPRESSURE RESTORES FLOW

By pressing or massaging neuro-lymphatic points, you stimulate the circulation of blood and lymph **and** encourage chi to move through the corresponding meridian. This dual action is why acupressure can relieve both physical pain and emotional stress at the same time.

For instance:

- Massaging a chest point may free tight breathing muscles, but it can also lighten feelings of sadness.
- Pressing abdominal points may relieve muscle aches, while also calming anxiety stored in the gut.

The Quick Fix Method sequences these points in a way that **restores flow across multiple meridians**, creating a whole-body balance effect in just a few minutes.

BALANCE AS THE GOAL

Pain is often the body's way of saying, *"Something is out of balance."* It may be a physical imbalance in posture, a chemical imbalance in digestion, an emotional imbalance from stress, or an energetic imbalance in chi. The Quick Fix Method doesn't treat disease or diagnose conditions—it simply helps bring the body back toward balance.

When balance is restored:

- Muscles relax.
- Pain signals quiet down.
- Emotions feel lighter.

- Energy feels more available for healing and daily living.

This is the deeper purpose of acupressure: not just to make the pain stop, but to reconnect you with the natural flow of life energy that supports health and harmony.

MODERN RESEARCH ON ACUPRESSURE

Although acupressure has been practiced for thousands of years as part of Traditional Chinese Medicine, modern science has only recently begun to explore its effects in measurable ways. Over the past few decades, researchers worldwide have conducted studies showing that acupressure can reduce pain, improve circulation, balance the nervous system, and even support emotional well-being.

PAIN RELIEF

Clinical studies have shown that stimulating acupressure points can significantly reduce pain:

- Patients with **chronic lower back pain** reported reduced discomfort and improved mobility after regular acupressure sessions.
- **Headache and migraine** sufferers experienced fewer and less intense episodes when using acupressure points between attacks.
- In hospitals, acupressure has been used successfully to reduce **post-surgical pain** and minimize the need for strong pain medications.

These outcomes suggest that acupressure is not just a traditional practice, but one with tangible physiological effects.

STRESS, ANXIETY, AND SLEEP

Modern research also shows acupressure's impact on the **autonomic nervous system**, which regulates stress and relaxation.

- Stimulation of specific points has been shown to reduce cortisol (the stress hormone) and promote calmness.
- Nursing studies report that patients who used acupressure techniques slept better and had lower levels of anxiety.
- This aligns with centuries-old knowledge that acupressure balances not only the body but also the mind and emotions.

CIRCULATION AND IMMUNITY

Research confirms what Dr. Chapman and others observed nearly a century ago: acupressure supports circulation and lymphatic flow. Improved circulation helps deliver oxygen and nutrients to tissues, while healthy lymphatic movement assists the immune system in clearing toxins. Some studies even suggest that regular acupressure can enhance immune resilience.

BRIDGING ANCIENT WISDOM AND MODERN EVIDENCE

While acupressure does not replace medical care, science increasingly validates what traditional healers have long understood:

- The body holds **built-in points of access** where simple touch can shift function.
- Relief often comes within minutes.
- Regular practice enhances not only symptom relief but also overall health and vitality.

The Quick Fix Method is grounded in this blend of **ancient practice and modern validation**. By focusing on key neuro-lymphatic points, it distills centuries of knowledge into a practical, evidence-supported method that anyone can learn.

The Five Types of Pain

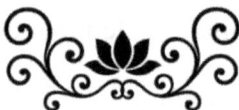

PHYSICAL PAIN

When most people think of pain, they think of the **physical kind**—the ache in the lower back, the throbbing of a sprained ankle, or the tension across tired shoulders. Physical pain is the body's most direct way of saying, *"Something isn't right."* It usually has a clear, measurable cause such as injury, strain, or inflammation.

Causes of Physical Pain

- **Injury or trauma** – cuts, sprains, fractures, or accidents.
- **Overuse or strain** – repetitive movements, poor posture, or lifting too much weight.
- **Inflammation** – arthritis, tendonitis, or irritated tissues.
- **Degeneration** – wear and tear of joints, muscles, or discs as we age.

Physical pain often shows up suddenly and demands attention, but it can also develop gradually through repeated stress on the body.

The Role of Quick Fix in Physical Pain

Acupressure, especially on neuro-lymphatic points, can help relieve physical pain in several ways:

- **Reduces muscle tension** by stimulating circulation in affected areas.
- **Supports lymphatic flow**, clearing toxins and easing inflammation.
- **Activates the nervous system's relaxation response**, calming pain signals.
- **Restores balance** to muscles and meridians, preventing compensation patterns that worsen discomfort.

For example:

- A tension headache may ease after massaging points along the chest and back that release neck and scalp muscles.
- Lower back pain may lessen when neuro-lymphatic points on the abdomen and thighs are stimulated, supporting spinal muscles.

Pain as a Guide

Physical pain is often the **most straightforward to interpret**—it tells you where the strain or injury is. Yet even here, there's wisdom. Rather than simply trying to silence the pain, you can use Quick Fix to work with your body:

- Noticing where tension collects.
- Releasing it through touch and breath.
- Allowing the body to reset itself.

Key Insight

Physical pain reminds us that the body is not a machine to be pushed endlessly—it is a living system that requires care, rest, and balance. Quick Fix offers a way to respect those signals while gently guiding the body back into harmony.

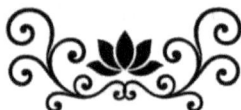

EMOTIONAL PAIN

Not all pain is physical. Sometimes the deepest aches are born from emotions—stress, grief, anger, fear, or heartbreak. While emotional pain may not leave visible marks on the body, it is just as real and often just as debilitating. The body and mind are not separate; what you feel emotionally often finds expression physically.

How Emotional Pain Shows Up in the Body

- Tight shoulders from carrying worry.
- An upset stomach when you're anxious.
- A heavy chest when you're grieving.
- Headaches during times of overwhelm.

Emotional experiences, especially unresolved ones, can be stored in the body's tissues. This is why people often describe emotions in physical terms: *"I feel a weight on my chest,"* or *"I have knots in my stomach."*

The Link Between Emotions and Pain

Science is now catching up to what traditional healing systems have long taught: emotions and physical health are deeply connected.

- Stress hormones like **cortisol and adrenaline** tighten muscles and increase pain sensitivity.
- Suppressed emotions can contribute to chronic pain syndromes.
- Traumatic experiences may become "locked" in the nervous system, reappearing as unexplained pain long after the event has passed.

The Role of Quick Fix in Emotional Pain

Acupressure can help release the physical grip of emotions on the body. By massaging neuro-lymphatic points, you:

- Ease muscle tension caused by emotional stress.
- Calm the nervous system, helping you shift from fight-or-flight to relaxation.
- Open energy pathways where feelings may have become blocked.

For example:

- Pressing points on the chest may release the weight of sadness or grief.
- Massaging abdominal points may calm anxiety stored in the gut.
- Stimulating back points may help the body "let go" of unprocessed frustration.

Pain as an Emotional Teacher

Emotional pain asks for acknowledgement. It says: *"Pay attention to what you're feeling. Don't bury it."* Quick Fix provides not just relief, but a gentle way to listen to emotions as they move through the body. Sometimes, pressing a point will bring a wave of feeling to the surface—a sign that energy is shifting and healing is taking place.

Key Insight

Emotional pain reminds us that healing is not only about the body—it is about the whole self. When you honor your emotions and give them space to be felt, the body responds with release, lightness, and balance.

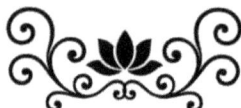

ENERGETIC PAIN

Sometimes pain does not arise from an injury, inflammation, or even a clear emotional trigger. Instead, it comes from **blocked or stagnant energy** in the body. This is known as **energetic pain**—discomfort that results when chi, or life-force energy, is unable to flow freely through the body's meridians and energy fields.

How Energetic Pain Feels

Energetic pain can be more subtle than physical or emotional pain, yet it is often just as disruptive. It may feel like:

- A heaviness or pressure in certain areas of the body.
- Tingling, numbness, or an odd "electric" sensation.
- Random aches that move or shift without explanation.
- Feeling drained, blocked, or "stuck" without an obvious cause.

Unlike physical pain, energetic pain often doesn't show up on X-rays, blood tests, or scans. Yet people know something is wrong because they *feel* it.

Where It Comes From

Energetic pain may be linked to:

- Blocked meridians that interrupt the flow of chi.
- Long-held stress or trauma is stored in the energy body.
- Environmental influences such as electromagnetic fields, toxins, or negative emotional atmospheres.
- Disconnection from one's natural rhythm or spiritual center.

Traditional Chinese Medicine, Ayurveda, and other healing systems have long recognized that when energy becomes imbalanced or stagnant, pain and illness follow.

The Role of Quick Fix in Energetic Pain

The Quick Fix Method is especially effective for energetic pain because it stimulates neuro-lymphatic points that connect directly to the meridians. When you press these points:

- Chi begins to move again, breaking up stagnation.
- The nervous system calms, allowing the body's energy to reset.
- Relief can often be felt within moments, as the "stuck" sensation shifts into flow.

For example:

- A feeling of heaviness in the chest may lift after stimulating points that open circulation and lung energy.
- Tingling or blocked sensations in the back may ease when abdominal points are massaged to balance spinal flow.

Key Insight

Energetic pain reminds us that we are more than muscles and bones—we are beings of energy. When energy flows smoothly, health and vitality are restored. Quick Fix gives you a simple way to unblock, balance, and harmonize your energy system so that pain no longer has to linger in hidden places.

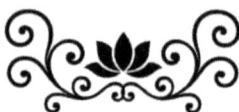

STRESS-INDUCED PAIN

Stress is one of the most common—and most underestimated—causes of pain in the modern world. Our bodies are designed to handle short bursts of stress, but when stress becomes chronic, it leaves its mark physically, emotionally, and energetically. This creates what is known as **stress-induced pain**.

How Stress Creates Pain

When you feel stressed, your body shifts into **fight-or-flight mode**. Stress hormones like cortisol and adrenaline surge through your system, preparing you to respond to danger. While this reaction is useful in emergencies, it becomes harmful when it is triggered daily by deadlines, finances, relationships, or constant pressure.

The results include:

- **Muscle tension** – shoulders, neck, and jaw tighten.
- **Restricted breathing** – shallow breaths reduce oxygen flow.
- **Headaches and fatigue** – from ongoing nervous system overload.

- **Lowered immunity** – leaving the body more vulnerable to illness.

Over time, these stress responses create a cycle: stress causes tension, tension causes pain, pain creates more stress—and the loop continues.

How Stress-Induced Pain Feels

- A "band" of tightness across the forehead.
- Burning or stiffness in the shoulders and upper back.
- A clenched jaw or grinding teeth at night.
- A sense of restlessness or exhaustion that doesn't go away with rest.

Unlike acute injuries, this pain often develops slowly, but it can become just as limiting as a physical injury.

The Role of Quick Fix in Stress-Induced Pain

Quick Fix interrupts the stress-pain cycle by calming both the body and the mind. By stimulating neuro-lymphatic points, you:

- Release muscular tension created by stress.
- Encourage deeper breathing, which lowers cortisol and soothes the nervous system.
- Shift the body from fight-or-flight into **rest-and-restore mode**.
- Restore circulation, leaving you with more energy and clarity.

For example:

- Applying Quick Fix before bedtime can reduce restlessness and allow for deeper sleep.

- Using the sequence during a stressful workday can dissolve the tension before it builds into a headache or neck pain.

Key Insight

Stress-induced pain is the body's way of saying: *"Slow down. Breathe. Reset."* By responding with Quick Fix, you not only relieve discomfort but also remind your body how to return to balance, even in the midst of life's demands.

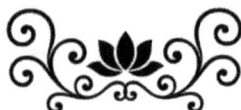

REFERRED / HIDDEN CAUSES OF PAIN

Sometimes pain appears in one part of the body, but its **true source lies elsewhere**. This is known as **referred pain**—when the nervous system "confuses" signals from one area and projects them into another. Hidden causes of pain can also be emotional, energetic, or postural patterns that aren't immediately obvious.

How Referred Pain Works

Nerves from different parts of the body often share the same pathways into the spinal cord. When the brain receives these overlapping signals, it may interpret discomfort as coming from the wrong location.

Examples include:

- **Heart pain** radiating into the left arm, shoulder, or jaw during a heart attack.
- **Gallbladder stress** is creating pain in the right shoulder blade.

- **Kidney problems** cause pain in the lower back or sides.
- **Sciatic nerve compression** sending shooting pain down the leg, even though the root is in the spine.

This type of pain can be confusing because it doesn't always respond when you treat the "spot that hurts."

Hidden Causes of Pain

Beyond referred pain, there are other hidden causes that often go unnoticed:

- **Postural imbalances** (slouching, uneven weight distribution) create strain elsewhere.
- **Emotional holding patterns**, such as grief stored in the chest or anger in the liver.
- **Energetic stagnation**, where blocked chi creates sensations that mimic muscular pain.
- **Old injuries or traumas** that healed on the surface but left behind lingering weakness or stress.

The Role of Quick Fix in Referred/Hidden Pain

Quick Fix cannot always eliminate the root cause of referred or hidden pain, but it can:

- Provide immediate relief by easing muscle tension surrounding the area.
- Improve circulation and energy flow, reducing the body's stress response.
- Help you **differentiate** between surface discomfort and deeper patterns that may need professional evaluation.

For instance:

- A tight shoulder from gallbladder stress may feel lighter after Quick Fix, but the underlying organ issue still requires care.
- Chronic sciatic pain may ease temporarily with Quick Fix, offering comfort while you address spinal alignment through therapy.

Key Insight

Referred and hidden pain remind us that the body is a network, not a set of isolated parts. Relief comes not just from pressing where it hurts, but from restoring balance throughout the system. Quick Fix provides you with a simple way to soothe discomfort in the moment, while giving you clarity about when deeper investigation may be needed.

Part II: The Quick Fix Method

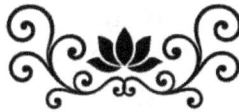

Your Hands as Healing Tools

The most powerful healing tools you will ever own are already with you—your **hands**. You don't need machines, needles, or expensive equipment to stimulate your body's natural healing ability. With a simple touch, gentle pressure, and clear intention, your hands can reduce pain, calm your nervous system, and restore balance in minutes.

THE HEALING POWER OF TOUCH

From the moment we are born, touch is one of the most fundamental ways we connect, comfort, and communicate. A mother's hand soothing a crying baby, a reassuring pat on the back, or a comforting hand placed on someone's shoulder—all of these gestures are forms of natural healing.

Science confirms what we instinctively know: touch stimulates the release of **endorphins**, the body's natural painkillers, and **oxytocin**, the hormone of trust and relaxation. It lowers blood pressure, reduces stress, and signals to the body that it is safe.

WHY HANDS ARE SO EFFECTIVE

Your hands are sensitive instruments, designed to both **sense** and **deliver** healing:

- **Sensitivity:** Your fingertips contain some of the body's highest concentrations of nerve endings, allowing you to feel subtle changes in tension, temperature, or energy flow.
- **Pressure and Movement:** Gentle massage of neuro-lymphatic points stimulates circulation and lymphatic flow, releasing blockages that contribute to pain.
- **Intention:** When you use your hands with focus and care, you direct not only physical touch but also healing energy into the body.

HEALING IS IN YOUR HANDS

You don't need special training to begin. As you follow the Quick Fix sequence, your hands will do the work naturally. With practice, you will become more aware of the sensations—heat, tingling, tenderness—that signal energy is moving and balance is being restored.

Remember:

- Your hands are **tools of awareness**—they help you listen to your body.
- Your hands are **tools of action**—they help you respond to pain in the moment.
- Your hands are **tools of empowerment**—they remind you that healing begins with you.

A SIMPLE BEGINNING

Before we dive into the full Quick Fix sequence, pause and try this:

1. Place one hand over your heart and the other on your abdomen.
2. Take three slow, deep breaths.
3. Notice the warmth, comfort, and sense of calm your own touch creates.

This is the essence of Quick Fix—using your hands to restore connection, relieve tension, and bring yourself back to balance.

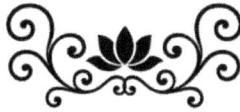

Touch, Pressure, and Intention

The Quick Fix Method is more than simply pressing points on the body. It is about *how* you touch, *how much* pressure you use, and the *intention* you bring to the process. These three elements work together to unlock the body's natural ability to release pain and restore balance.

THE LANGUAGE OF TOUCH

Touch communicates directly with the nervous system. A light, caring touch signals safety and calms stress, while firm, steady pressure stimulates circulation and helps release tension. Both have their place.

When applying Quick Fix:

- **Gentle Touch** reassures the body and helps you locate sensitive areas.
- **Moderate Pressure**—firm but comfortable—stimulates the neuro-lymphatic points without creating pain.

- **Massage-like Movements**—small circles or steady rubbing—help break up stagnation and encourage lymphatic flow.

The goal is never to force, but to encourage release.

FINDING THE RIGHT PRESSURE

A common question is: *How hard should I press?* The answer: **just enough to feel tender, but not so much that it hurts.**

Think of it as polishing, not pounding.

- If you press too lightly, the body may not respond.
- If you press too hard, the body tenses up in defense, blocking the flow.
- The right pressure feels a little sore, but also relieving— as though you are reaching an itch you didn't know you had.

Always listen to your body. Sensitivity may change day by day, or even point by point.

THE POWER OF INTENTION

Perhaps the most important element of Quick Fix is the one you cannot see: **your intention.**

When you approach the practice with focus and care, you send a clear message to your body: *"I am listening. I am ready to release this pain. I trust my body's ability to heal."*

Research in psychoneuroimmunology (the study of how thoughts and emotions influence health) shows that intention and mindset affect the body's chemistry. A calm, positive focus enhances the effects of acupressure and accelerates healing.

PUTTING IT TOGETHER

Each time you place your hands on a neuro-lymphatic point, remember that you are combining three forces:

1. **Touch** – the physical connection.
2. **Pressure** – the stimulation that activates release.
3. **Intention** – the energy that directs the body toward healing.

Together, they transform a simple sequence of movements into a powerful tool for relief and renewal.

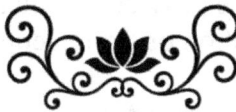

Safety and Contraindications

The Quick Fix Method is designed to be **safe, gentle, and accessible** for most people. However, like any healing practice, there are times when extra caution is needed. Understanding when and how to use Quick Fix ensures that you get the most benefit while protecting your health.

GENERAL SAFETY GUIDELINES

- **Comfort first:** Pressure should never cause sharp or severe pain. Tenderness at the points is normal, but if it feels unbearable, ease up.
- **Breathe naturally:** Holding your breath can create tension. Keep your breathing slow and relaxed as you work through the sequence.

- **Go slowly:** If you are new to acupressure, begin with a lighter touch and shorter sessions. Gradually increase as your body becomes more comfortable.
- **Hydrate:** Drinking water after a session supports lymphatic flow and helps the body flush out toxins released during the sequence.
- **Rest if needed:** If the points feel unusually sore or you feel fatigued afterward, give your body time to integrate before repeating the practice.

WHEN TO USE CAUTION

Quick Fix is not a substitute for medical care. Always consult your doctor or healthcare provider if you are uncertain about your condition. Use caution or avoid acupressure if you have:

- **Serious or unexplained pain** – especially sudden chest pain, severe abdominal pain, or pain radiating into the arm or jaw.
- **Injuries or open wounds** in the areas where pressure points are located.
- **Pregnancy** – some acupressure points may stimulate uterine contractions; check with a qualified practitioner before using.
- **Severe circulatory or lymphatic conditions** such as blood clots or uncontrolled lymphedema.
- **Infectious illness or fever** – the body needs rest and medical care, not stimulation.
- **Cancer, heart conditions, or other chronic diseases** – acupressure may be supportive but should always be cleared with your healthcare provider first.

THE ROLE OF QUICK FIX

Quick Fix is meant to **support** your health, not replace professional treatment. It works best as a complementary practice—reducing pain, calming the nervous system, and restoring balance while you continue with any necessary medical care.

Think of Quick Fix as part of your **self-care toolkit**—a method that empowers you to respond to discomfort safely, quickly, and naturally. When used responsibly, it can bring relief and comfort to daily life, while leaving space for doctors and healthcare professionals to play their vital role when needed.

***

Use Quick Fix as part of your self-care, but remember: **professional medical care is essential when needed.** If you are uncertain about your symptoms or condition, always check with your healthcare provider.

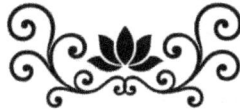

The Quick Fix Pain Relief Chart

HOW TO READ THE CHART

The Quick Fix Pain Relief Chart is your roadmap. It shows you the exact neuro-lymphatic points used in the Quick Fix sequence, organized so you can easily follow along and apply them to yourself or guide someone else. Think of it as a visual shortcut that keeps the method clear, simple, and repeatable.

KEY FEATURES OF THE CHART

- **Body Diagrams:** The chart highlights specific areas on the front and back of the body where neuro-lymphatic points are located.
- **Numbered Sequence:** Each point is marked with a number or letter so you know the exact order to follow.
- **Point Descriptions:** Some versions of the chart include short notes or keywords to remind you of the location or function of each point.
- **Left to Right Symmetry:** Many points appear on both sides of the body; unless noted otherwise, you will massage them on both the left and right.

HOW TO FOLLOW THE CHART

1. **Start at the Top:** The sequence is usually designed to begin at the upper body and move downward, supporting a natural flow of circulation and energy.
2. **Follow the Numbers:** Move in order from one point to the next. This ensures balance and avoids overstimulating any single area.
3. **Apply Pressure or Massage:** At each point, use firm but comfortable pressure. Massage for about **5–10 seconds** or until you feel a slight release or warmth.
4. **Breathe:** With each point, take a slow, deep breath. Breathing amplifies the effect of the stimulation and calms the nervous system.
5. **Repeat on Both Sides:** Unless the chart indicates otherwise, work the point on both the left and right sides of the body.
6. **Complete the Sequence:** Once all points are covered, take a moment to notice how your body feels—lighter, looser, or freer.

Why I Begin at Kidney 24

Although the Quick Fix Chart is designed as a sequence, I have found myself naturally beginning at **Kidney 24**, which overlaps with an important point on the **Governing Vessel (Du Mai)**. This point, located just below the collarbone near the sternum, is a vital place where physical, emotional, and energetic systems intersect.

In Traditional Chinese Medicine, **Kidney energy** represents vitality, resilience, and the deep reserves that sustain life. The **Governing Vessel** is often described as the body's "control channel," influencing the flow of energy along the spine and throughout the nervous system.

By starting here, a few things happen:

- **Physical:** The chest opens, breathing deepens, and circulation improves right from the beginning.
- **Emotional:** This area is closely linked to feelings of safety and release—making it an ideal entry point for calming stress.
- **Energetic:** Stimulating this spot activates both Kidney reserves and Governing Vessel flow, setting the tone for balance throughout the rest of the sequence.

Interestingly, K24 is also positioned very close to the **neuro-lymphatic drainage reflexes for the lungs**. These reflex points, mapped by Dr. Frank Chapman, are located in the second and third intercostal spaces near the sternum—only a couple of finger widths away. In addition, the body's main lymphatic return channel, the thoracic duct, empties into the venous system just above the clavicle, making this entire region a major hub for both circulation and drainage.

This means that when you stimulate Kidney 24, you are not only activating a powerful meridian point but also influencing lymphatic flow and respiratory balance at the same time.

For me, beginning with Kidney 24 feels like pressing the **"reset button"** for the body's energy. It prepares the system to respond more effectively to the rest of the Quick Fix points.

While you can follow the chart in its entirety from start to finish, don't be surprised if you, too, feel drawn to begin here. The body often knows where it most needs attention, and this point can act as a powerful doorway into the Quick Fix experience.

TIPS FOR USING THE CHART EFFECTIVELY

- **Keep It Visible:** Print or place the chart somewhere you can see easily while practicing—by a mirror, on the wall, or flat on a table.
- **Practice by Feel:** Over time, you'll rely less on the chart and more on your body's feedback. Sensitivity, tenderness, or warmth will guide you to the right points.
- **Use it as a Reference, Not a Test:** The chart is there to support you, not overwhelm you. If you miss a point or forget a step, that's okay. Simply return to the sequence and continue.
- **Notice Patterns:** As you practice, you may find certain points feel consistently tender. This can be a clue to where your body is holding stress or imbalance.

The chart is your **compass**, but your body is the true guide. With practice, the Quick Fix sequence will become second nature, and you'll be able to follow your body's signals with confidence—whether or not you have the chart in front of you.

QUICK FIX PAIN RELIEF ACUPRESSURE CHART

Video Link
https://youtu.be/dQGnHNaW3_w

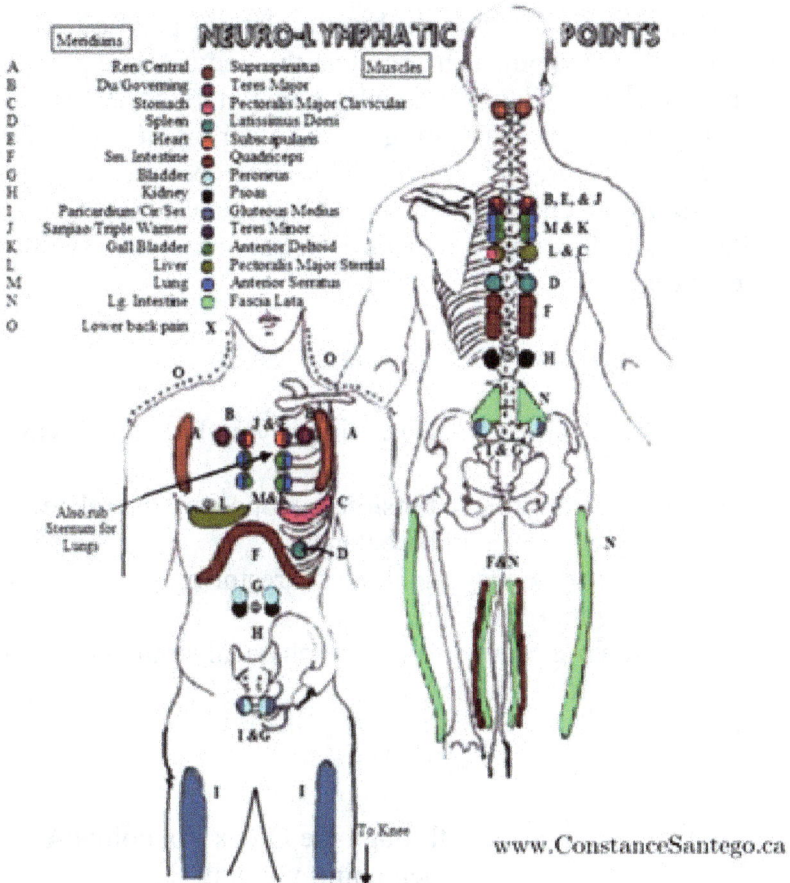

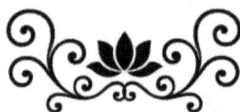

INTRODUCTION TO THE
NEURO-LYMPHATIC POINTS

The Quick Fix Method works by stimulating specific **neuro-lymphatic reflex points** mapped on the body. These points were first described by Dr. Frank Chapman in the 1930s, and later integrated into kinesiology and Touch for Health by Dr. George Goodheart and Dr. John Thie. Each point corresponds to a **meridian** (an energy pathway in Traditional Chinese Medicine) and to a **muscle group**, linking physical structure with energetic flow.

By massaging these points, you are:

- **Activating circulation** – improving blood and lymph flow.
- **Releasing muscle tension** – supporting the related muscle to relax and rebalance.
- **Clearing energy blockages** – restoring the flow of chi through the meridians.
- **Relieving pain** – both from physical strain and from stress stored in the body.

HOW TO USE THIS SECTION

This guide will walk you through the Quick Fix points **A through O** in detail. For each point, you will learn:

- **The letter** (as shown on the chart).
- **The meridian** it is linked to.
- **The associated muscle** that benefits from stimulation.
- **The color code** from the chart is for quick reference.

- **The function/benefit** – what happens when you stimulate the point.
- **Quick Fix insight** – how this point contributes to reducing pain and restoring balance.

As you read, remember: you don't need to memorize every detail. The chart gives you the roadmap, and your body gives you feedback. This section simply deepens your understanding so you can feel more confident as you practice.

NEURO-LYMPHATIC POINTS

	Meridians		Muscles
A	Ren/Central	●	Supraspinatus
B	Du/Governing	●	Teres Major
C	Stomach	●	Pectoralis Major Clavicular
D	Spleen	●	Latissimus Dorsi
E	Heart	●	Subscapularis
F	Sm. Intestine	●	Quadriceps
G	Bladder	○	Peroneus
H	Kidney	●	Psoas
I	Paricardium/Cir/Sex	●	Gluteous Medius
J	Sanjiao/Triple Warmer	●	Teres Minor
K	Gall Bladder	●	Anterior Deltoid
L	Liver	●	Pectoralis Major Sternal
M	Lung	●	Anterior Serratus
N	Lg. Intestine	○	Fascia Lata
O	Lower back pain	X	

NEURO-LYMPHATIC POINT A
– REN/CENTRAL MERIDIAN

Meridian: Ren (Central)
Associated Muscle: *Supraspinatus*
Color on Chart: Red

Location: Both sides—starting at the bony front of the shoulder joint, trace down along the outer edge of the breast on both sides of the chest.

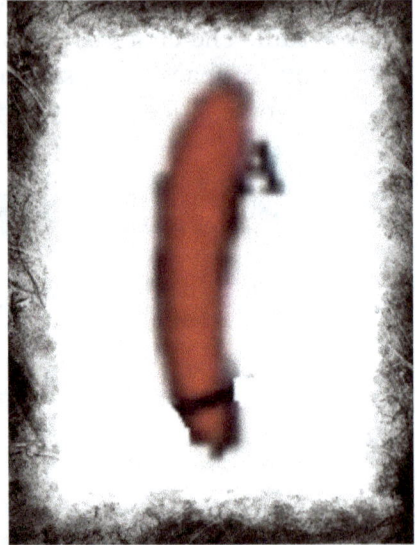

Function/Benefit:
The Ren (Central) meridian is sometimes called the "Sea of Yin," responsible for nourishing the entire body's Yin energy (fluids, cooling, restoring). Stimulating these points helps balance the upper body, opens the chest, and supports breathing.

The *Supraspinatus muscle* assists in lifting the arm and stabilizing the shoulder joint. Tightness here is often linked with shoulder or upper back discomfort. By activating the Ren/Central points, you relieve shoulder tension, improve posture, and restore a sense of centeredness.

Quick Fix Insight:
Point A serves as a grounding start to the sequence. Massaging here awakens the body's central channel, supporting emotional calm and physical alignment.

Quick Note:

These points lie over the **sternal lymphatic reflex zones**, which support drainage from the chest and lungs. Stimulating Point A therefore combines energetic alignment with improved circulation and lymph flow in the upper body.

NEURO-LYMPHATIC POINT B
– DU/GOVERNING MERIDIAN

Meridian: Du (Governing)
Associated Muscle: *Teres Major*
Color on Chart: Dark Red

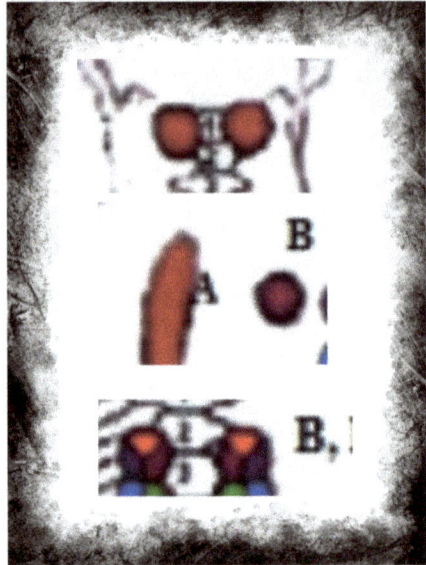

Location: Cervical-C1, then both sides, and both front and back—

Front points: Between ribs 2–3, about 2–3 inches lateral from the sternum (breastbone).

Back points: Between thoracic vertebrae T2–T3, approximately 1 inch to each side of the spine.

Function/Benefit:
The **Du (Governing) meridian** is often referred to as the "Sea of Yang," running along the midline of the back and influencing the entire spine and nervous system. Stimulating this point on the chest helps activate circulation through the Governing Vessel, encouraging balance between the body's Yin and Yang energies.

The *Teres Major muscle* assists with arm movements such as internal rotation and pulling the arm back (like when reaching behind you). Tension here can create shoulder stiffness, limited range of motion, or upper back discomfort. Working Point B helps relax this muscle and improve shoulder mobility.

Quick Fix Insight:
Point B is like a "switch" for resetting the spine and shoulders. Stimulating it encourages energy to flow up the Governing Vessel, supporting posture, spinal balance, and overall vitality. Many people feel their breathing deepen and their upper back relax within moments.

Quick Note on Kidney 24 & Lymphatic Drainage:

Although Point B is mapped to the **Du/Governing meridian** and the **Teres Major muscle**, it also lies very close to **Kidney 24 (K24)** and the **neuro-lymphatic drainage reflexes** for the lungs.

Stimulating this area not only supports spinal alignment and shoulder function but also:

- Opens the chest for deeper breathing.
- Encourages **lymphatic drainage** through the thoracic duct region.
- Relieves congestion and tension that may present as chest tightness or stress.

This makes Point B especially powerful, as it works at the intersection of **energy flow, muscle release, and lymphatic detoxification**.

NEURO-LYMPHATIC POINT C
– STOMACH MERIDIAN

Meridian: Stomach (ST)
Associated Muscle: *Pectoralis Major (Clavicular portion)*
Color on Chart: Pink

Location: One front **point**—On
the **left side of the chest**, between
ribs 5–6, running from the nipple
line inward toward the sternum
(breastbone).

Back point: Between the thoracic
vertebrae **T5–T6**, approximately
one inch to each side of the
spine.

Function/Benefit:
The **Stomach meridian** governs
digestion and vitality. It is closely
tied to the body's ability to transform nourishment into usable
energy, and imbalances often appear as fatigue, digestive upset,
or worry.

The *Pectoralis Major (clavicular fibers)* helps bring the arm
forward and across the chest. Tension or weakness here
contributes to rounded shoulders, chest tightness, or restricted
arm movement. Stimulating Point C relieves chest tension,
improves posture, and supports digestive health.

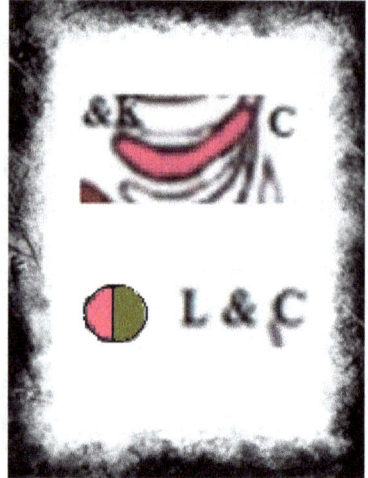

Quick Fix Insight:
Point C is often tender in those who carry stress in the chest or who struggle with digestive issues. Massaging here lightens the chest, softens worry, and helps restore grounding.

Quick Note:
This point sits near the **anterior thoracic lymphatic reflexes** connected with both digestion and lung function. Stimulating it may help ease bloating, reduce chest congestion, and calm stress-related digestive upset.

NEURO-LYMPHATIC POINT D
– SPLEEN MERIDIAN

Meridian: Spleen (SP)
Associated Muscle: *Latissimus Dorsi*
Color on Chart: Green

Location: Front point:
Between ribs **7–8** near the costal
cartilage, most often on the **left
side**. This spot may feel like a
slight **depression** or tender
notch.

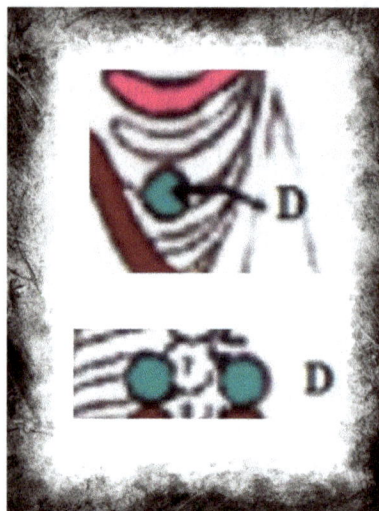

Back point: Between thoracic
vertebrae **T7–T8**, about **1 inch**
to each side of the spine.

Function/Benefit:
The **Spleen meridian** is central
to digestion, nutrient absorption, and immune function. In
Traditional Chinese Medicine, it is linked with transformation
and transportation—the ability to convert food into usable
energy and distribute it throughout the body. Emotionally, the
spleen is tied to worry and overthinking.

The *Latissimus Dorsi* is a large back muscle involved in
pulling, reaching, and stabilizing the spine and shoulders.
Tightness here can contribute to back strain, shoulder
discomfort, and limited upper body mobility.

Stimulating Point D can:

- Relieve tension through the ribcage and back.
- Support digestion and immune resilience.
- Release worry or mental heaviness stored in the body.

Quick Fix Insight:
Point D is a powerful "bridge" point: it links the body's core muscles with emotional grounding. Working here often brings a sense of stability, ease in the back, and relief from the mental fog of overthinking.

Quick Note:
These lateral chest points lie near **neuro-lymphatic reflex zones for digestion and lymph drainage**. By stimulating Point D, you are not only helping the Latissimus Dorsi relax but also encouraging lymphatic movement through the trunk, which supports detoxification and reduces inflammation-related pain.

NEURO-LYMPHATIC POINT E
– HEART MERIDIAN

Meridian: Heart (HT)
Associated Muscle: *Subscapularis*
Color on Chart: Deep Red

Location: Front point: Between ribs **2–3**, close to the **sternum (breastbone)**, bilaterally.

Back point: Between thoracic vertebrae **T2–T3**, about **1 inch** to each side of the spine.

Function/Benefit:
The **Heart meridian** governs circulation, emotional balance, and vitality. In Traditional Chinese Medicine, the heart is considered the "Emperor" of the body—housing the spirit (Shen) and influencing clarity of thought, joy, and calmness. Imbalances often show up as anxiety, restlessness, or shallow breathing.

The *Subscapularis muscle*, located beneath the shoulder blade, helps rotate the arm inward and stabilize the shoulder. Tension or weakness here is often linked with shoulder pain, frozen shoulder, or restricted arm movement.

Stimulating Point E can:

- Ease chest tightness and support healthy circulation.
- Calm the nervous system and reduce anxiety.
- Relieve shoulder restriction by supporting the Subscapularis balance.

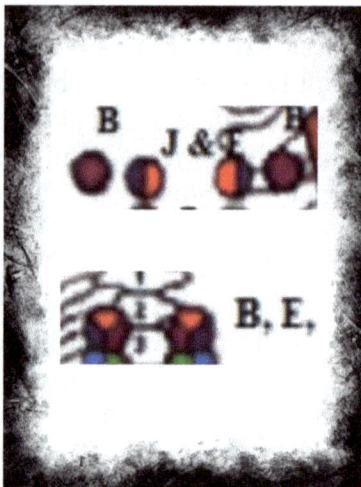

Quick Fix Insight:
Point E is a **heart-opener** in every sense: physically, it opens the chest and shoulders; emotionally, it lightens heaviness and restores calm. Many people notice an immediate sense of relief here, as if "taking a weight off the chest."

Quick Note:
Point E lies near **neuro-lymphatic reflexes for both the heart and lungs,** making it especially valuable for releasing tension in the chest and improving circulation. Stimulating this area not only helps reduce shoulder pain but also supports emotional release, particularly in cases of stress, grief, or anxiety stored in the chest.

NEURO-LYMPHATIC POINT F
– SMALL INTESTINE MERIDIAN

Meridian: Small Intestine (SI)
Associated Muscle: *Quadriceps (Rectus Femoris portion)*
Color on Chart: Brown

Location: Front points: Along
the lower ribcage, between ribs **8–
11**, near the costal cartilage,
tracing the curve at the bottom of
the rib cage.

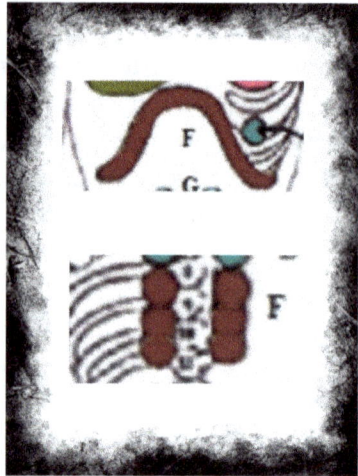

Back points: Between thoracic
vertebrae **T8–T12**, approximately
1 inch to each side of the spine.

Function/Benefit:
The **Small Intestine meridian** is
responsible for separating "clear from turbid"—absorbing what
the body needs and eliminating what it does not. Emotionally,
this meridian is tied to discernment, clarity, and decision-
making. Imbalances can manifest as bloating, poor digestion, or
indecisiveness.

The *Rectus Femoris* (one of the quadriceps muscles) plays a
major role in hip flexion and knee extension. Weakness or
tightness here can contribute to knee pain, hip strain, or postural
imbalance.

Stimulating Point F can:

- Support digestive absorption and reduce abdominal
  discomfort.
- Relieve tension in the front of the thighs and hips.
- Encourage clarity and emotional decisiveness.

Quick Fix Insight:
Point F often feels tender for people who carry digestive stress or mental overwhelm. By massaging here, you not only ease abdominal tension but also help "sort out" both physical digestion and mental clutter.

Quick Note:
These abdominal points lie near **Chapman's neuro-lymphatic reflexes for the intestines**, meaning they also stimulate lymphatic drainage of the gut. This makes Point F doubly effective for reducing bloating, calming stomach upset, and improving posture by releasing lower abdominal tension.

NEURO-LYMPHATIC POINT G
– BLADDER MERIDIAN

Meridian: Bladder (BL)
Associated Muscle: *Peroneus*
Color on Chart: Light Blue

Location: Front points: On the abdomen, **to either side of the navel** (belly button), and along the **upper edges of the pubic bone**.

Back points: Over the **posterior superior iliac spines (PSIS)** — the prominent knobs on the back of the hip bones — at the level of **L5** in the lumbar spine.

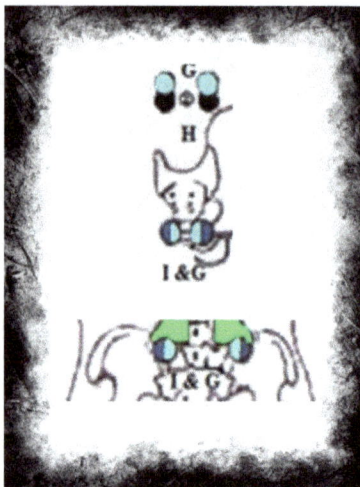

Function/Benefit:

The **Bladder meridian** is the longest pathway in Traditional Chinese Medicine, running along the entire back of the body. It influences the nervous system, spine, and the release of stored tension. Emotionally, the Bladder meridian is connected with fear and the ability to "let go."

The *Peroneus muscles* (longus and brevis) stabilize the ankle and support balance during walking. Imbalances here can show up as ankle instability, shin pain, or gait issues.

Stimulating Point G can:

- Improve ankle stability and relieve lateral leg pain.
- Support spinal balance and reduce lower back strain.
- Release deep-seated tension linked with fear and stress.

Quick Fix Insight:
Point G is a **structural and emotional release point**. Working here often eases both lower back tension and ankle/leg discomfort, while also calming the nervous system.

Quick Note:
The lateral lower leg overlaps with **neuro-lymphatic reflexes tied to circulation and pelvic/lumbar function**. Stimulating Point G promotes lymphatic return from the legs, reduces swelling or fatigue, and relieves lumbar strain indirectly.

NEURO-LYMPHATIC POINT H
– KIDNEY MERIDIAN

Meridian: Kidney (KI)
Associated Muscle: *Psoas*
Color on Chart: Black

Location: Front points: About
1 inch to the sides of the navel
and **1 inch above** it.

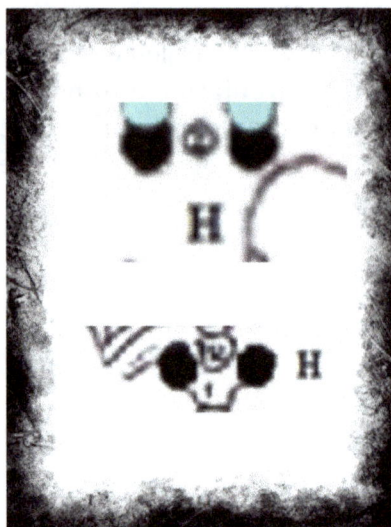

Back points: Between **T12 and
L1**, just below the last ribs,
approximately **1 inch** to each
side of the spine.

Function/Benefit:
The **Kidney meridian** is
considered the "root of life" in
Traditional Chinese Medicine.
It governs energy reserves, vitality, reproductive health, and the
balance of water in the body. Emotionally, it is linked with fear,
willpower, and resilience.

The *Psoas muscle* is a deep core muscle that connects the spine
to the legs, essential for posture, walking, and stability. Chronic
tightness here often causes low back pain, hip problems, and
feelings of "holding stress in the gut."

Stimulating Point H can:

- Release deep-seated abdominal and hip tension.
- Strengthen core stability and reduce lower back strain.
- Restore energy reserves and calm deep-seated fears.

Quick Fix Insight:
Point H is often tender but profoundly relieving. Massaging here feels like unlocking a hidden storehouse of tension. Many people report immediate ease in the lower back and hips, as well as a sense of inner calm and renewed vitality.

Quick Note:
These points are also close to **neuro-lymphatic reflexes for the kidneys and adrenals**. Stimulating Point H supports detoxification, relieves adrenal stress, and boosts both physical and emotional endurance—making it one of the most powerful points in the Quick Fix sequence.

NEURO-LYMPHATIC POINT I
– CIRCULATION/SEX MERIDIAN

Meridian: Circulation/Sex (Pericardium, PC)
Associated Muscle: *Gluteus Medius*
Color on Chart: Blue

Location: Front points: Along the **upper edge of the pubic bones**, bilaterally.

Back points: Over the **posterior superior iliac spines (PSIS)** — the prominent knobs of the hip bones — at the level of **L5** in the lumbar spine.

Function/Benefit:
The **Circulation/Sex (Pericardium) meridian** protects the heart and governs intimacy, circulation, and emotional connection. Imbalances may show up as poor circulation, pelvic congestion, or emotional withdrawal.

The *Gluteus Medius muscle* stabilizes the pelvis during walking, standing, and hip movement. Weakness here often contributes to hip instability, lower back pain, or gait imbalance.

Stimulating Point I can:

- Support pelvic balance and relieve lower back/hip strain.
- Encourage healthy circulation in the pelvic region.
- Enhance emotional openness and intimacy.

Quick Fix Insight:
Point I is a **pelvic stabilizer**. Massaging here often relieves tension across the hips and low back, while also lightening emotional blockages tied to vulnerability or disconnection.

Quick Note:
This point corresponds with **neuro-lymphatic reflexes for pelvic drainage**. Stimulating it improves lymphatic flow in the lower abdomen and pelvis, easing congestion, menstrual discomfort, or tension patterns that radiate into the hips and low back.

NEURO-LYMPHATIC POINT J
– TRIPLE WARMER MERIDIAN

Meridian: Triple Warmer (San Jiao, TW/SJ)
Associated Muscle: *Teres Minor*
Color on Chart: Purple

Location: Front points:
Between **ribs 2–3**, close to the
sternum (breastbone).

Back points: Between **T2–T3**,
about **one inch lateral** to each
side of the spine.

Function/Benefit:
The **Triple Warmer meridian**
(also called San Jiao) governs the
body's temperature regulation,
metabolism, and stress response. Energetically, it acts as the
"general" of the immune system, mobilizing defenses when the
body is under pressure. Emotionally, it is strongly tied to
anxiety, overdrive, and survival mode.

The *Teres Minor muscle* helps with external rotation of the
shoulder and stabilizes the arm. Tightness or weakness here
often contributes to shoulder pain, rotator cuff imbalance, or
difficulty lifting the arm overhead.

Stimulating Point J can:

- Release shoulder tightness and restore mobility.
- Calm the stress response and reduce feelings of being
  "on edge."
- Support immune and adrenal balance.

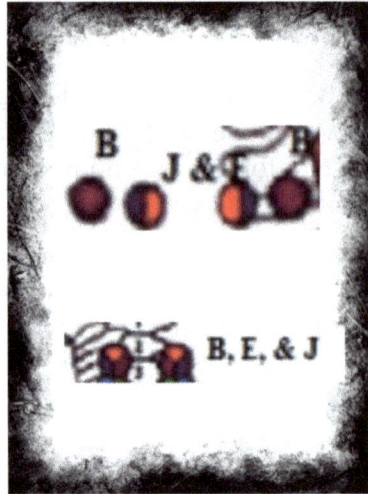

Quick Fix Insight:
Point J is one of the most important points for modern life. It helps the body "switch off" from fight-or-flight mode and return to a calmer state, while also improving shoulder function. Many people notice an immediate sense of relaxation in both the body and mind.

Quick Note:
This region lies near **neuro-lymphatic reflexes for immune and adrenal support**. Massaging Point J not only relieves shoulder discomfort but also encourages lymphatic drainage in the upper chest, supporting resilience against stress and immune challenges.

NEURO-LYMPHATIC POINT K
– GALLBLADDER MERIDIAN

Meridian: Gallbladder (GB)
Associated Muscle: *Anterior Deltoid*
Color on Chart: Dark Green

Location: Front points:
Between **ribs 3–4 and 4–5,**
close to the sternum
(breastbone).

Back points: Between **T3–T4
and T4–T5,** about **one inch
lateral** to each side of the
spine.

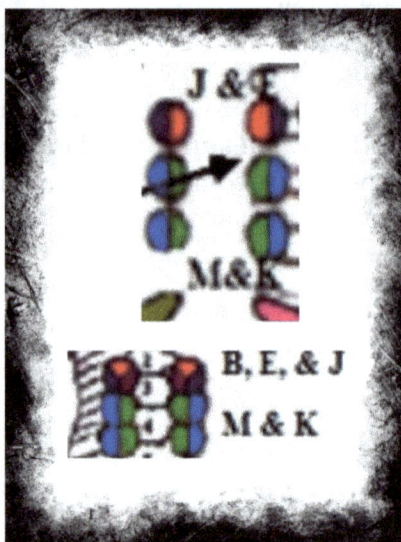

Function/Benefit:
The **Gallbladder meridian**
governs decision-making, courage, and the smooth flow of Qi
throughout the body. In TCM, it is linked with flexibility—both
physically (joints) and emotionally (adaptability). Imbalances
often show up as stiffness, indecision, or irritability.

The *Anterior Deltoid muscle* raises the arm forward and plays a
role in stabilizing the shoulder joint. Weakness or tightness here
can limit lifting motions, cause shoulder pain, and contribute to
poor posture.

Stimulating Point K can:

- Release tension in the front of the shoulder.
- Support healthy decision-making and emotional clarity.
- Improve mobility and stability in the arms and upper
  body.

Quick Fix Insight:
Point K is especially helpful for people who feel "weighed down" by indecision or who carry stress in their shoulders. Stimulating it restores both **shoulder freedom** and **mental clarity**—making it easier to move forward, physically and emotionally.

Quick Note:
The shoulder region also corresponds with **lymphatic drainage pathways for the arms and upper chest**. Working Point K supports healthy circulation and lymphatic flow in the arms, helping relieve shoulder stiffness while reducing fluid buildup or fatigue in the upper extremities.

NEURO-LYMPHATIC POINT L
– LIVER MERIDIAN

Meridian: Liver (LV)
Associated Muscle: *Pectoralis Major (Sternal fibers)*
Color on Chart: Moss Green

Location: Front point: On the right side only, between **ribs 5–6,** running from the **nipple line to the sternum (breastbone).**

Back point: At the level of **T5–6,** about **one inch to the right side of the spine.**

Function/Benefit:
The **Liver meridian** governs detoxification, blood storage, and the smooth flow of Qi throughout the body. Emotionally, it is linked to anger, frustration, and the ability to plan and take decisive action. Imbalances may show up as irritability, digestive upset, eye strain, or tension in the chest and ribcage.

The *Pectoralis Major (sternal fibers)* draws the arm across the body and helps stabilize the chest and shoulders. Tightness here often leads to rounded shoulders, shallow breathing, or chest restriction.

Stimulating Point L can:

- Open the chest and reduce muscular tension across the front of the body.
- Support detoxification and circulation of blood and lymph.
- Release frustration or irritability stored in the chest.

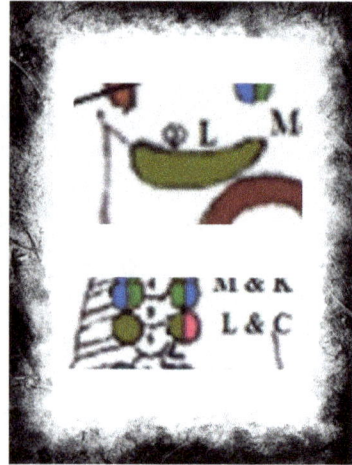

Quick Fix Insight:
Point L is both **physical and emotional release**—loosening up tight chest muscles while also creating a sense of emotional spaciousness. Many people feel a "lightening" effect here, as if letting go of frustration and reclaiming calm.

Quick Note:
This region lies over **neuro-lymphatic reflexes for liver function and chest drainage**. Stimulating Point L not only helps posture and breath but also supports detoxification and lymphatic clearance—making it one of the most important Quick Fix points for restoring energy.

NEURO-LYMPHATIC POINT M
– LUNG MERIDIAN

Meridian: Lung (LU)
Associated Muscle: *Serratus Anterior*
Color on Chart: Cobalt Blue

Location: Front point: Between ribs 3–4 and 4–5, close to the sternum (breastbone).

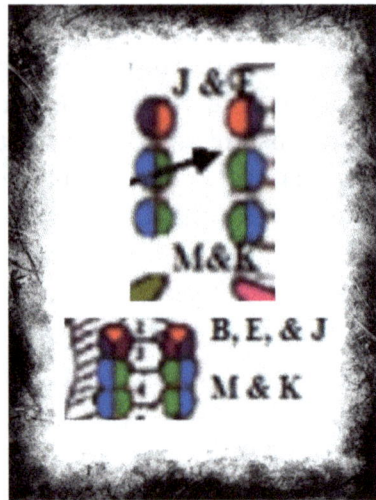

Back point: Between **T3–4 and T4–5**, about **one inch to each side of the spine**.

Function/Benefit:
The **Lung meridian** governs breath, energy (Qi), and the immune system. In Traditional Chinese Medicine, the lungs are said to "control Qi and respiration" and are strongly connected to the emotions of grief and sadness. Imbalances can show up as shallow breathing, fatigue, low immunity, or tightness across the chest.

The *Serratus Anterior muscle* helps move and stabilize the shoulder blades, playing a key role in breathing and arm mobility. Weakness or tightness here can contribute to shoulder pain, poor posture, and restricted breathing capacity.

Stimulating Point M can:

- Expand lung capacity and support deeper breathing.
- Relieve chest and rib tension.
- Support immune health and emotional release of grief or heaviness.

Quick Fix Insight:
Point M is often described as a **"breath release" point**.
Massaging here creates a sense of expansion through the ribs,
making it easier to breathe fully. On an emotional level, it can
feel like lifting a weight off the chest, allowing space for relief
and renewal.

Quick Note:
This point is located near **neuro-lymphatic reflexes for the
lungs** and helps clear congestion in the respiratory system.
Stimulating Point M not only improves breathing but also
encourages lymphatic drainage through the thoracic region,
supporting both physical and emotional cleansing.

NEURO-LYMPHATIC POINT N
– LARGE INTESTINE MERIDIAN

Meridian: Large Intestine (LI)
Associated Muscle: *Tensor Fasciae Latae / Fascia Lata*
Color on Chart: Neon Green

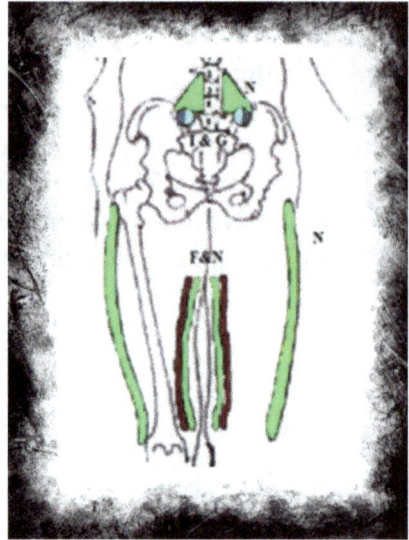

Location: Front point: From the **top of the thigh bone (femur)** down to about **one inch below the kneecap**, tracing along the entire **outside (lateral side) of both legs**.

Back point: In the **triangular region between L2, L4, and the highest crest of the hip bone (iliac crest)**.

Function/Benefit:
The **Large Intestine meridian** is linked to elimination and letting go—both physically (waste removal, detoxification) and emotionally (releasing grief, stagnation, or old burdens).

The *Tensor Fasciae Latae* (part of the fascia lata) stabilizes the hip and knee through the iliotibial (IT) band. Tightness here can create lateral leg pain, hip stiffness, or knee tracking issues.

Stimulating Point N helps to:

- Relieve tension along the IT band and outer thigh.
- Support hip and knee alignment.
- Improve elimination, digestion, and detoxification.
- Release stored stress or emotional "holding on."

Quick Fix Insight:
Point N is excellent for people with **hip or knee discomfort**, as well as those who carry tension in the outer thighs from walking, running, or sitting long hours. On the energetic side, it's a powerful point for **"letting go"**—whether of waste, stress, or grief.

Quick Note:
Because of its placement, this point strongly influences **lymphatic drainage of the pelvis and lower extremities**. Activating it not only eases physical tightness but also helps reduce **leg swelling, heaviness, and circulation issues**.

AREA O
– SHOULDER REFLEX FOR LOWER BACK RELEASE

Meridian: *None directly* (structural/neurological reflex)
Associated Muscle Relationship: *Opposites – Shoulders ↔ Lower Back*
Color on Chart: XXXXXXXX's

Location: Across the tops of the shoulders (trapezius area), where a gentle pinch or squeeze can be applied bilaterally.

Function/Benefit:
Point O works on the principle of **reciprocal muscle relationships**: stimulating one muscle group can release tension in its opposite. In this case, the shoulders and lower back share a reflex connection. By applying pressure or a light pinch across the shoulders, the **lower back muscles are encouraged to relax**.

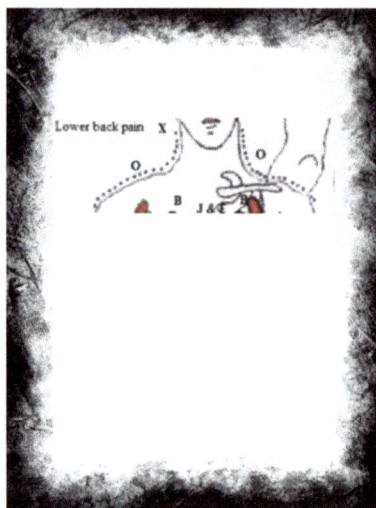

This point is especially useful when the lower back feels tight, spasmodic, or locked up. Instead of working directly on the painful area, you use the shoulders as a **reflex key** to "switch off" the tension in the back.

Stimulating Point O can:

- Relieve lower back pain by releasing the opposite shoulder muscles.
- Loosen tightness in the trapezius, easing shoulder and neck stress.

- Provide rapid pain relief without having to press directly on the sore lower back.

Quick Fix Insight:
Point O is a **surprise release point**. Many people don't expect that working on the shoulders can unlock the lower back, but it often produces immediate and dramatic results. It's a perfect example of how the body is interconnected, and how pain is not always solved by treating the area where it shows up.

Quick Note:
Though not linked to a traditional meridian, this reflex fits the same logic as **neuro-lymphatic and applied kinesiology balancing methods**—where tension in one region can be corrected through its paired or opposing muscle group. By stimulating the shoulders, you are not just relaxing the upper body but also activating a chain reaction that relieves the spine and lumbar region.

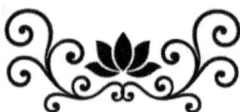

STEP-BY-STEP GUIDE TO THE QUICK FIX SEQUENCE

The Quick Fix Sequence is designed to clear neuro-lymphatic reflex points in a logical order, helping restore balance across the whole body. While you can start anywhere on the chart if intuition guides you, following the sequence ensures a full reset.

1. Begin at Point A – Ren/Central Meridian

- Rub along the midline of the chest to awaken the central channel, calm the system, and ground your energy.
- This serves as your "starting switch."

2. Move to Point B – Du/Governing Meridian

- Stimulate the upper chest near K24.
- This opens the lungs, improves breathing, and activates lymphatic drainage.

Think of this as pressing the body's "reset button."

3. Work Down the Sequence (Points C–M)

- **C – Stomach**: Balance digestion, relieve stomach tension.
- **D – Spleen**: Boost immunity, support circulation.
- **E – Heart**: Open chest, reduce anxiety, support cardiac energy.
- **F – Small Intestine**: Improve absorption, relieve abdominal tightness.
- **G – Bladder**: Release lower back, hip, and hamstring tension.
- **H – Kidney**: Support vitality, lower back, and fluid balance.

- **I – Circulation/Sex (Pericardium)**: Release pelvic tension, balance hormones.
- **J – Triple Warmer (San Jiao)**: Regulate stress and energy distribution.
- **K – Gall Bladder**: Relieve side-body tension, improve decision-making clarity.
- **L – Liver**: Clear frustration, aids detoxification.
- **M – Lung**: Deepen breath, strengthen immunity.

4. Stimulate Point N – Large Intestine

- Massage along the sides of the thighs (Tensor Fasciae Latae).
- This promotes elimination, supports detox, and helps the hips/knees release strain.

5. Finish with Point O – Shoulder Pinch (Lower Back Release)

- Use a light pinch across the tops of both shoulders.
- This reflexively releases tension in the **lower back** while encouraging full-body relaxation.

How to Use the Sequence

1. **Rub firmly but comfortably** — enough pressure to stimulate circulation without causing pain.
2. **Follow the flow** — A through O, unless your body guides you elsewhere.
3. **Take deep breaths** as you work through the points to enhance oxygenation and relaxation.
4. **Reassess your pain** when you finish. Often, pain shifts or reduces immediately.
5. **Repeat daily if needed** — especially for chronic discomfort, stress, or fatigue.

Quick Fix Insight:
Think of this sequence as a **reset circuit for your body's energy and lymphatic flow.** It clears congestion, supports detoxification, balances meridians, and relaxes the muscles all in one short routine. Many people notice results in minutes.

OR

STEP-BY-STEP GUIDE TO THE QUICK FIX SEQUENCE

The Quick Fix begins at **Kidney 24 (K24)**, located between the 2nd and 3rd ribs, a few inches from the sternum. This point overlaps with the **Du/Governing meridian** and is also close to lymphatic drainage reflexes. Starting here helps to **reset the body's energy system, open the chest, and prepare the whole sequence for deeper release.**

1. Start at Point B – K24 / Du-Governing

- **Front:** Between ribs 2–3, 2–3 inches from the sternum.
- **Back:** Between T2–3, one inch from each side of the spine.
- Stimulating this point clears chest congestion, awakens lymphatic flow, and connects the Governing channel with Kidney energy.

Think of it as the "ignition switch" for the Quick Fix.

2. Move to Point A – Ren/Central Meridian

- Located along the midline of the chest.
- Awakens the central channel, grounds Yin energy, and supports calm.
- Together, A & B balance the **front (Ren) and back (Du) vessels**.

3. Continue Through the Sequence (C–M)

- **C – Stomach:** Front digestion reset; back at T5–6 for upper abdomen relief.
- **D – Spleen:** Left rib area; supports immunity and circulation.
- **E – Heart:** Upper chest, T2–3; calms stress and strengthens heart energy.
- **F – Small Intestine:** Along rib curve; aids nutrient absorption and abdominal release.
- **G – Bladder:** Navel/hip area & sacrum; frees hamstrings, hips, and lower back.
- **H – Kidney:** One inch above/sides of navel; replenishes vitality and fluid balance.
- **I – Circulation/Sex (Pericardium):** Pubic bone/hips; pelvic energy and hormone balance.
- **J – Triple Warmer:** Chest ribs 2–3; regulates stress and overall energy.
- **K – Gall Bladder:** Ribs 3–5; side-body relief, clears tension.
- **L – Liver:** Right ribs 5–6; detox and emotional release.
- **M – Lung:** Ribs 3–5; strengthens breath, clears grief.

4. Point N – Large Intestine (Fascia Lata)

- **Front:** Outside of thighs, hip to below knee.
- **Back:** Triangle between L2, L4, and the top of the hip bone.
- Encourages elimination, clears stagnation, and relieves hip/knee tension.

5. Point O – Shoulder Reflex for Lower Back Release

- Light pinch across the shoulders.
- This "opposite reflex" eases lower back pain and completes the circuit.

How to Use This Sequence

1. **Start at K24 (Point B)** — always first.
2. Move to Point A, then continue down through **C–M, then N, ending at O.**
3. Use **firm but comfortable pressure** or circular rubbing for 20–30 seconds per point.
4. **Breathe deeply** with each point, allowing tension to release.
5. Reassess pain level when finished; repeat daily if needed.

Quick Fix Insight:
By beginning at **K24**, you activate one of the most powerful neuro-lymphatic reflexes, often used as a "switch-on" point in applied kinesiology. From there, the sequence flows through all major meridians, lymphatic drainage zones, and muscle resets — making it a whole-body tune-up in just minutes.

IF YOU CAN'T REACH THE POINTS ON YOUR BACK

Some of the Quick Fix points are located along the spine or upper back, which can be challenging to reach without assistance. Don't worry — there are simple solutions:

- **Ask for Help:** A partner, friend, or family member can rub or press the back points for you while you guide them on the location and pressure.
- **Use a Door Frame:** Stand with your back against a doorway and lean into the frame at the level of the points. Rock gently side to side, "scratching" the area like a bear to stimulate the reflexes.
- **Try a Massage Tool:** a tennis ball, foam roller, or handheld massage stick can be used to press into the points when you need extra reach.
- **Do What You Can:** Even stimulating the front points alone often produces strong results, since the Quick Fix works through reflex pathways that connect front and back.

Quick Fix Insight:
You don't have to be perfect with technique to get results. Your body responds to touch, intention, and movement — whether it's your hands, a helper, or a doorframe.

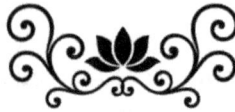

The Quick Fix Routine

PREPARATION & BREATH

Before you begin the Quick Fix sequence, it's important to prepare your body and mind. This step ensures your nervous system is calm, your focus is present, and your energy is ready to shift.

1. Find Your Space
The beauty of Quick Fix is that you can do it *anywhere* — while sitting in a chair, standing by your desk, lying in bed, or even in the bathroom first thing in the morning. All you need is a moment of focus and your own two hands.

2. Center Yourself
Close your eyes briefly and bring your awareness inward. Notice how your body feels. Where do you sense tension? Rate your pain on a scale of 1 to 10. This simple check-in becomes your baseline for measuring change.

3. Breathe with Intention
Take three slow, deep breaths:

- **Inhale** through the nose, filling the chest and abdomen.
- **Hold** gently for a pause.
- **Exhale** through the mouth, releasing tension with your breath.

This activates the parasympathetic nervous system — the body's "rest and repair" mode — making the Quick Fix sequence more effective.

4. Set Your Intention
Quietly affirm what you want from this session:

- Relief from a specific pain.
- Greater ease in your body.
- Emotional calm or mental clarity.

Your intention directs the flow of energy, much like setting a compass before a journey.

5. Ready to Begin
Once grounded, bring your hands to the starting point — **Kidney 24 (Point B)**. This little ritual takes less than a minute but primes your entire system for deeper release and balance.

Quick Fix Insight:
The breath is your first medicine. Before your fingers touch a single point, your lungs, diaphragm, and nervous system are already opening the pathways for healing. And remember — this doesn't require a meditation cushion or special setup. Some of the best Quick Fix sessions happen in everyday spaces, even on the edge of your bed or while sitting on the toilet in the morning.

VIEW THE YOUTUBE VIDEO:
By Dr. Constance Santego
Demonstration of the Quick Fix
HTTPS://YOUTU.BE/DQGNHNAW3_W

APPLYING THE SEQUENCE

The Quick Fix sequence is designed to be flexible — you can begin at any point on the body and still receive benefit. However, I have found that starting at **Point B (Kidney 24 / Du-Governing)** consistently gives the best results. This point, located just under the collarbone between the 2nd and 3rd ribs, acts like a reset switch for the body's energy, opening the chest, engaging lymphatic drainage, and preparing the nervous system for balance.

How to Apply the Sequence:

1. **Choose Your Starting Point**
    o   If you're new, follow the chart from **A through O** for a full-body reset.
    o   If you're experienced, trust your intuition — sometimes the body "calls out" the point it needs most.
    o   For me, I almost always begin with **Point B (K24)** because it sets the tone for the rest of the sequence.
2. **Apply Firm, Gentle Pressure**
    o   Use the tips of your fingers to rub or massage each point.
    o   Apply steady, comfortable pressure — firm enough to feel circulation, but never painful.
    o   Work each point for **5–15 seconds** (or longer if especially tender).
3. **Follow the Flow**
    o   Move through the points in order (A–O), or create your own sequence based on your needs.
    o   Breathe deeply as you go, letting your exhale release tension from the body.

4. **Reassess Your Pain**
   o After completing the sequence, pause. Move (shimmy):
      ▪ Has the pain shifted?
      ▪ Is the intensity lower?
      ▪ Do you feel more relaxed or open?
5. **Repeat if Needed**
   o If pain remains above a 2–3 on your pain scale, repeat the sequence a second time.
   o For persistent or recurring pain, daily practice builds lasting results.
   o **If the pain (number) does not change**, seek professional help. In my experience, this often indicates a **structural issue** such as a bone being out of alignment, which may require the attention of a **chiropractor**. In some cases, it could also signal the need for **medical evaluation by a doctor** to rule out other causes.

Quick Fix Insight:
Your body is wise — sometimes the most effective sequence is the one it asks for in the moment. While the full A–O flow is powerful, don't be afraid to experiment. And if you're not sure where to begin, **Point B (K24)** is always a reliable place to start.

Self-care is powerful, but it works best when paired with professional support when needed. The Quick Fix method helps address many sources of muscular and energetic pain — but if pain persists, your body may be asking for a deeper adjustment or medical care.

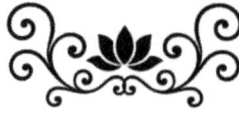

REASSESSING PAIN LEVELS

An important part of the Quick Fix routine is learning to **check in with your body before and after the sequence**. This gives you real-time feedback on whether the points are helping and guides your next steps.

1. Establish Your Baseline

- Before beginning, rate your pain on a scale of **1 to 10**, with **1 = very mild** and **10 = the worst pain imaginable.**
- Note where you feel it: Is it sharp, dull, heavy, or tight? Is it localized or spreading?

2. Check During the Sequence

- As you move through the points, pause at the halfway mark (around Point H) and notice:
    - Has the pain shifted in location?
    - Has the intensity dropped, even slightly?
    - Do you feel warmth, tingling, or emotional release?
    These are all signs the Quick Fix is working.

3. Reassess at the End

- After finishing the sequence, repeat the movement that originally caused discomfort.
- Re-rate your pain from 1–10. Often, people report a **2–5 point drop** after just one round.

4. Decide What's Next

- If pain has reduced but not fully cleared, repeat the sequence a second time.
- If pain is **gone or significantly improved**, celebrate — your body responded beautifully.
- If pain remains unchanged after two rounds, it may be structural (a joint or bone issue) or medical in nature. At this point, it's wise to seek professional care from a **chiropractor** (for alignment) or a **medical doctor** (to rule out underlying conditions).

Quick Fix Insight:
Pain is not just a nuisance — it's your body's **language**. Even if the pain moves, shifts, or changes quality (from sharp to dull, or from one spot to another), it means your body is responding. Listening carefully helps you know when to keep going and when to get support.

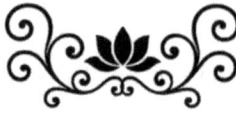

REPETITION & MUSCLE MEMORY

One of the reasons people often need multiple chiropractic adjustments or bodywork sessions is because of **muscle memory**. A chiropractor may realign the spine or reset a joint, but if the muscles surrounding that area are still tense, weak, or patterned with old habits, they can easily pull the bones right back out of place. This is why follow-up treatments are usually required.

The Quick Fix method helps address this problem directly. By stimulating **neuro-lymphatic reflex points**, you aren't just working on the bones — you're helping the muscles **release their stored tension and reset their firing patterns.** When the muscles relax, they stop tugging the bones back out of alignment.

This means:

- **Adjustments last longer.** Your chiropractor's work is supported by the Quick Fix routine.
- **Fewer treatments are needed.** Because the muscles are learning new patterns, your body holds balance more naturally.
- **You take back control.** Instead of waiting for the next appointment, you have a tool in your hands to keep your body in alignment.

Why Repetition Matters

Just like learning a new skill or habit, your muscles and nervous system need repetition to "reprogram." Each time you run the Quick Fix sequence, you're training your body to let go of old holding patterns and create new ones:

- The **first time**, you may feel immediate relief.
- With **consistent practice**, your body learns to respond faster and more deeply.
- Over time, the Quick Fix becomes a kind of "muscle reset button" that your body remembers and responds to automatically.

Quick Fix Insight:
Think of it this way: if chiropractic is about **resetting the structure**, Quick Fix is about **retraining the software** (your muscles and nervous system). Together, they create lasting results.

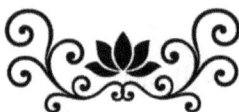

Quick Fix for Common Issues

Headaches & Migraines

Headaches and migraines are among the most common types of pain people face — and they can stop life in its tracks. While there are many causes (stress, muscle tension, dehydration, hormones, or even structural misalignments), two points in the Quick Fix sequence are especially powerful for bringing relief:

- **Gallbladder Point K (Front ribs 3–5 / Back T3–5):**
  The Gallbladder meridian runs along the sides of the head and temples — a classic migraine pathway. Stimulating Point K helps relieve shoulder and neck tension that often triggers headaches, while also clearing stuck energy from the Gallbladder channel.
- **Large Intestine Point N (Outer thighs & lumbar triangle):**
  The Large Intestine meridian travels up through the face and sinuses, making it another key channel in headache relief. Stimulating Point N helps release fascia tension in the hips and legs, which surprisingly can ease pressure patterns that radiate upward into the neck and head.

How to Apply the Quick Fix

1. Start at **Point B (K24)** to open the chest and reset circulation.
2. Move to **Point K (Gallbladder)** and massage firmly, front and back.

3. Stimulate **Point N (Large Intestine)** along the outside thighs and lumbar triangle.
4. Breathe deeply, allowing tension to drain downward and out of the head.
5. Reassess — many people feel a lightening of pressure in minutes.

Extra Support

- **Hydration:** Drink a glass of water after completing the sequence. Dehydration is a hidden trigger in many headaches.
- **Neck & Shoulder Release:** Combine with gentle neck stretches or a warm compress for added relief.
- **Stress Check-In:** Headaches are often the body's way of saying, "slow down." Pair this Quick Fix with a few minutes of rest or quiet breathing.

Quick Fix Insight:
Headaches often represent **upward-rising tension** — too much energy pooling in the head. The Quick Fix sequence works by **pulling energy back down through the body, releasing congestion** from the neck, shoulders, and head.

NECK & SHOULDER TENSION

Neck and shoulder tightness is one of the most common pain patterns today — whether it's caused by long hours at a desk, driving, stress, or poor posture. It may feel like stiffness, heaviness, or radiating discomfort into the head, upper back, or arms.

The Quick Fix approach works by releasing both the **local tension points** and the **opposite stabilizers** in the hips and buttocks. This dual approach prevents the "tug of war" that keeps tension locked in.

Key Points for Relief:

- **Point A – Ren/Central Meridian (Chest midline & outer breast):**
  Opens the central channel and supports posture, which directly reduces forward head and rounded shoulders.
- **C1 Reflex Points (base of the skull):**
  Part of point A. Gentle pressure applied at the base of the skull, specifically around the atlas vertebra (C1), where the head bends, helps release suboccipital tension that often drives neck stiffness and headaches.
- **Point B – Du/Governing (K24 area, ribs 2–3 / T2–3):**
  Opens the chest, resets the upper spine, and engages lymphatic drainage — a powerful "reset" for shoulder girdle tension.
- **Point E – Heart (Ribs 2–3 near sternum / T2–3):**
  Releases emotional stress and chest tightness that pulls the shoulders forward.
- **Point G – Bladder (Abdomen/pubic bones / PSIS at L5):**
  Supports spinal alignment from the lower back up — often neck and shoulder tension begins in pelvic misalignment.

- **Point I – Circulation/Sex (Hips & buttocks, Gluteus Medius):**
  Reflex-opposite release. Massaging the hips and buttocks relaxes the shoulder girdle by balancing its opposing muscles.
- **Point K – Gallbladder (Ribs 3–5 / T3–5):**
  Clears tension along the sides of the neck and shoulders — especially helpful when tightness radiates up toward the temples.

How to Apply the Quick Fix

1. Start with **Point B (K24)** to open the chest.
2. Stimulate **Points A, E, and K** across the chest and upper back.
3. Massage the **C1 reflex points** at the base of the skull.
4. Balance the system by massaging **Point I (hips/buttocks)** and **Point G (pelvic reflexes)**.
5. Reassess neck and shoulder movement; repeat if needed.

Extra Support

- Apply gentle heat across the upper back and neck before starting.
- For tension headaches, combine with **Point L (Liver)** to help release stress and irritability.
- Always check posture — correcting forward head or slouched shoulders is key to long-term relief.

Quick Fix Insight:
Neck and shoulder pain rarely lives in isolation. By combining **local points (A, B, E, K)** with **opposite stabilizers (G, I)**, you release the entire tension chain from pelvis to skull — unlocking relief in minutes.

BACK PAIN

Back pain is one of the most common reasons people seek help, whether from a doctor, chiropractor, or therapist. It can range from dull stiffness to sharp spasms that make movement nearly impossible. Because the back is connected to nearly every movement we make, even small imbalances can create big discomfort.

The Quick Fix method approaches back pain by addressing **local reflexes** (points directly tied to the spine and core stability) and **opposite or supportive points** that help the back release more effectively.

Key Points for Relief:

- **Point H – Kidney (Front 1" up and out from navel / Back T12–L1):**
  Core stabilizer via the *Psoas*. Releasing here reduces deep lower back tension and replenishes Kidney energy — often depleted in people with chronic pain.
- **Point N – Large Intestine (Outer thighs & lumbar triangle):**
  Balances the pelvis and fascia lata, relieving pressure on the lumbar spine. Tight IT bands often pull on the hips, which translates into lower back pain.
- **Point O – Shoulder Reflex for Lower Back:**
  A light pinch across the tops of the shoulders reflexively relaxes the lumbar muscles. This "opposite release" can give immediate relief when the lower back feels locked.

Additional Supportive Points:

- **Point G – Bladder (Front pubic/abdominal area & Back PSIS at L5):**
  Stabilizes the sacrum and hips, easing lower spine strain.

- **Point B – Du/Governing (K24 area / T2–3):**
  Supports spinal alignment from above, helping the whole chain balance.
- **Point A – Ren/Central (chest midline):**
  Improves posture and prevents the chest from collapsing forward — a major hidden cause of low back compression.

How to Apply the Quick Fix

1. Begin with **Point B (K24)** to activate energy flow.
2. Stimulate **Point H (Kidney/Psoas)** for deep lumbar release.
3. Massage **Point N (outer thighs and lumbar triangle)** to balance pelvic stability.
4. Use a light **shoulder pinch at Point O** to reflexively relax the lower back.
5. Add **Point G (Bladder reflexes)** if pain feels sacral or hip-related.
6. Reassess your pain level and repeat if needed.

Extra Support

- Apply gentle heat to the lower back before the sequence.
- Pair with **hip flexor stretches** or a simple knee-to-chest stretch afterward.
- Hydrate well — dehydration often worsens disc and joint pain.
- For persistent back pain, chiropractic or medical support may be needed if structural issues are involved.

Quick Fix Insight:
Back pain is often a **whole-body issue**, not just a local problem. By combining **deep stabilizer points (H)**, **pelvic/leg release points (N, G)**, and the surprising **opposite reflex (O)**, the Quick Fix sequence creates both immediate relief and long-term resilience.

STRESS & ANXIETY

Stress and anxiety affect not just the mind but the whole body. They tighten muscles, restrict breathing, raise blood pressure, and disrupt digestion. Left unchecked, they can also amplify physical pain. The Quick Fix routine calms both the **nervous system** and the **emotional body** by activating points that release tension, deepen breath, and reset energy balance.

Key Points for Relief:

- **Point E – Heart (Ribs 2–3 near sternum / Back T2–3):**
  Opens the chest, eases emotional strain, and calms the *Shen* (spirit/heart-mind). Excellent for racing thoughts and tightness in the chest.
- **Point M – Pericardium (Ribs 3–5 near sternum / Back T3–5):**
  Protects the heart and regulates circulation. Often tender in people under constant stress. Releasing here feels like "taking a weight off the chest."
- **Point J – Triple Warmer (Ribs 2–3 near sternum / Back T2–3):**
  Balances the body's stress response (fight-or-flight). Activating this point signals the system to "stand down," bringing a wave of calm.
- **Point A – Ren/Central (Chest midline & outer breast):**
  Grounds Yin energy, brings emotional stability, and restores centeredness.
- **Point B – Du/Governing (K24 / T2–3):**
  A natural starting point. Helps regulate the nervous system and improve breathing under stress.

How to Apply the Quick Fix

1. Start with **Point B (K24)** to open the chest and calm the nervous system.
2. Move to **Point E (Heart)** and **Point M (Pericardium)** for chest and emotional release.
3. Add **Point J (Triple Warmer)** to regulate the stress response.
4. Finish with **Point A (Ren/Central)** to restore calm and grounding.
5. Take three slow, deep breaths before reassessing.

Extra Support

- Pair the sequence with **visualization**: imagine exhaling stress as gray mist leaving the body.
- Use calming aromatherapy (lavender, frankincense, bergamot) during the sequence.
- Practice daily for prevention, not just during stressful moments.

Quick Fix Insight:
Stress and anxiety are signs that the body's energy has shifted into **overdrive**. By stimulating these points, you invite the body back into its natural state of balance — calm, open, and at ease.

FATIGUE & LOW ENERGY

Fatigue shows up when the body's reserves are drained — whether from stress, poor sleep, overwork, or underlying health issues. Unlike simple tiredness, this kind of low energy lingers and can affect focus, mood, and resilience. The Quick Fix sequence helps by stimulating points that **boost circulation, free blocked energy, and restore vitality**.

Key Points for Renewal:

- **Point H – Kidney (Front near navel / Back T12–L1):**
  The Kidney meridian is considered the body's "battery." Stimulating here replenishes deep reserves of energy, calms exhaustion, and supports adrenal function.
- **Point M – Lung (Ribs 3–5 near sternum / Back T3–5):**
  Expands breathing capacity and boosts oxygen intake — key to quickly replenishing energy.
- **Point D – Spleen (Ribs 7–8 cartilage / Back T7–8):**
  Supports digestion and nutrient absorption. When the spleen is sluggish, energy feels heavy, and fatigue lingers.
- **Point B – Du/Governing (K24 area / T2–3):**
  Acts as an "ignition switch." In addition to rubbing, try **light, rhythmic pounding with the fingertips** across this area to energize circulation and awaken the nervous system.

How to Apply the Quick Fix

1. Begin with **light pounding at Point B (K24)** — 10–15 gentle taps to wake up circulation.
2. Stimulate **Point H (Kidney)** to strengthen core vitality.
3. Move to **Point M (Lung)** for breath expansion.
4. Add **Point D (Spleen)** to support digestion and energy production.

5. Take 3 energizing breaths — inhale deeply, exhale
    forcefully through the mouth.

Extra Support

- Pair the Quick Fix with a glass of water — dehydration
  is a hidden cause of fatigue.
- Practice **morning and mid-afternoon** when energy dips
  most.
- Combine with uplifting aromatherapy (peppermint,
  citrus, rosemary) to stimulate alertness.
- If fatigue is chronic or unexplained, consult a healthcare
  provider to rule out underlying issues.

Quick Fix Insight:
Fatigue is often not just about needing more rest — it's about
blocked or depleted energy. By activating these points,
especially with a stimulating technique like light pounding at
Point B, you can spark your system back into flow and reclaim
your vitality in minutes.

Part III: Living Pain-Free

Synergistic Healing: Blending Quick Fix with Other Tools

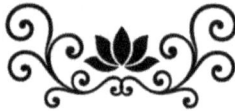

AROMATHERAPY

Aromatherapy is one of the simplest and most powerful ways to enhance the Quick Fix method. Essential oils work directly through the **olfactory system**, which connects to the brain's limbic center — the area responsible for emotions, memory, and stress response. This means that the right oil can quickly shift your mood, calm anxiety, or energize the body, complementing the relief you create through acupressure.

How Aromatherapy Enhances Quick Fix:

- **Pain Relief:** Oils such as lavender, peppermint, and eucalyptus help relax muscles and reduce tension.
- **Emotional Balance:** Frankincense, bergamot, and clary sage calm the nervous system and ease anxious thoughts.
- **Energy Boost:** Citrus oils like orange, lemon, and grapefruit invigorate the senses and pair beautifully with the fatigue-relief points in the sequence.

- **Circulation & Detox:** Rosemary, ginger, and juniper berry stimulate circulation and support lymphatic drainage — the very system Quick Fix activates.

Simple Ways to Combine Aromatherapy with Quick Fix:

1. **Topical Application:** Dilute 2–3 drops of essential oil in a carrier oil (like coconut or jojoba) and apply over the chest or back points you are working on. This enhances the effect of rubbing neuro-lymphatic reflexes.
2. **Inhalation:** Place a drop or two in your palms, rub together, and cup your hands over your nose. Inhale deeply before starting the sequence to calm the mind.
3. **Diffusion:** Use a diffuser in your practice space. A calm scent creates an environment of safety and relaxation, which helps the nervous system respond more quickly.

Quick Fix Insight:
When you stimulate a neuro-lymphatic point and inhale a supportive oil at the same time, you create a **multi-sensory healing experience** — the body responds physically, emotionally, and energetically, making the release deeper and more lasting.

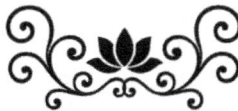

REFLEXOLOGY

Reflexology works on the principle that the entire body is mirrored in the feet, hands, and ears. By stimulating specific reflex zones, you can influence organs, glands, and systems throughout the body. When combined with the Quick Fix sequence, reflexology adds another layer of support for releasing tension and restoring balance.

How Reflexology Enhances Quick Fix:

- **Pain Relief:** Working on reflex points for the spine, neck, or shoulders in the feet can amplify the results of acupressure on the body.
- **Stress Reduction:** Foot reflexology naturally calms the nervous system, grounding the body and enhancing the parasympathetic "rest and repair" response.
- **Circulation & Detox:** Reflex stimulation promotes blood and lymph flow, complementing the neuro-lymphatic massage points of Quick Fix.
- **Whole-Body Support:** By addressing both the acupressure points and their corresponding foot reflexes, you create a more complete system of healing.

Simple Ways to Combine Reflexology with Quick Fix:

1. **Start at the Feet:** Before doing Quick Fix, gently massage the foot reflexes for the spine (along the inner edge of the foot) and kidneys (center of the sole). This primes the body for release.
2. **During the Sequence:** If you are focusing on a specific issue — for example, headaches — stimulate the reflex for the head and sinuses on the toes while also working Point K (Gallbladder) and Point N (Large Intestine).
3. **Finish with Grounding:** After Quick Fix, rub the reflex points for the solar plexus (center of the foot below the ball). This encourages full relaxation and integration of the release.

Quick Fix Insight:
Reflexology is like opening the body's "circuit breakers" through the feet. When paired with Quick Fix, you connect both **direct neuro-lymphatic points** and their **reflex counterparts**, doubling the effectiveness of your self-care routine.

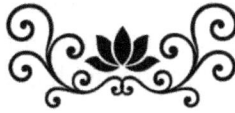

VISUALIZATION & BREATHWORK

Your breath is one of the most powerful tools for healing — it bridges body and mind, physical and energetic systems. When combined with visualization, breathwork becomes a way to **direct energy, calm the nervous system, and amplify the effects of the Quick Fix sequence.**

How Visualization & Breathwork Enhance Quick Fix:

- **Pain Release:** Visualizing tension melting or draining away while exhaling helps the body let go faster.
- **Energy Flow:** Breath brings oxygen and life force (Qi/Prana) into the body, carrying it along the meridians you are stimulating.
- **Emotional Balance:** Guided imagery calms anxious thoughts, making the release of emotional pain smoother.
- **Integration:** Breath and imagery anchor the Quick Fix results, so the body remembers the new, relaxed state.

Simple Ways to Combine Visualization & Breathwork with Quick Fix:

1. **Cleansing Breath:** As you rub each point, inhale through your nose, then exhale through your mouth as if "blowing out" the pain. Imagine dark smoke leaving your body with each exhale.
2. **Color Visualization:** Assign a healing color to each breath. For example, breathe in a cool blue light at Point E (Heart) to calm anxiety, or a golden light at Point H (Kidney) to restore vitality.

3. **Directional Breathing:** Imagine inhaling energy into the point you're working, then exhaling it down through the body and out through the hands or feet — creating a sense of flow and release.
4. **Anchor with Intention:** At the end of the sequence, close your eyes, take three deep breaths, and visualize your body glowing with balance and ease.

Quick Fix Insight:
Your imagination isn't just in your head — it's a healing tool. When you combine the **physical touch of Quick Fix points** with the **inner guidance of breath and imagery**, you align body, mind, and spirit for deeper and longer-lasting results.

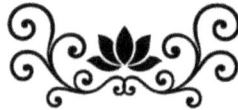

The Mind-Body Connection

Emotions Stored in the Body

Our bodies are not just physical structures; they are also living records of our experiences. Every stress, every loss, every unspoken word leaves an imprint. When emotions are not expressed or resolved, they often take up residence in the body as **tension, pain, or chronic discomfort.**

- **Neck and Shoulders:** Often carry the "weight of responsibility," showing up as stiffness when life feels overwhelming.
- **Lower Back:** Commonly reflects worries about safety, finances, or feeling unsupported.
- **Chest/Heart Area:** Holds grief, heartbreak, and unexpressed emotions of love or loss.

- **Hips and Pelvis:** Store fear, trauma, and emotions tied to intimacy and creativity.
- **Stomach and Gut:** The seat of worry and anxiety, often manifesting as tightness, indigestion, or knots.

The Quick Fix sequence is not just about rubbing muscles or stimulating points — it's about **unlocking stored emotion** and allowing it to move. Sometimes a point may feel more tender than expected, or you may notice emotions rising as you work on it. This is the body's way of saying: *"I'm ready to let this go."*

How to Work with Emotional Release During Quick Fix:

1. **Notice Tenderness:** If a point feels unusually sore, pause. Breathe into it. Ask yourself, *What might I be holding here?*
2. **Allow Emotion:** Tears, sighs, yawns, or even laughter are natural releases. Let them flow without judgment.
3. **Use Intention:** As you massage, silently repeat affirmations like, *"I release what no longer serves me,"* or *"I am safe and supported."*
4. **Finish with Integration:** Place your hands over your heart or abdomen when you're done. Take three slow breaths to signal completion and peace.

Quick Fix Insight:
Pain is often the body's way of expressing what the mind and heart could not. By stimulating neuro-lymphatic points, you're not only releasing tension but also giving stored emotions a chance to move, transform, and heal.

RELEASING PAIN AS RELEASING ENERGY

At its core, pain is energy — a signal that something is blocked, stuck, or demanding attention. Whether physical, emotional, or spiritual, pain represents energy that has stopped flowing freely. When you engage with the Quick Fix sequence, you are not only addressing muscles or reflex points, but also **moving stagnant energy** out of the body.

Think of it this way:

- **Physical Pain** is often energy locked in muscle tension or inflammation.
- **Emotional Pain** is energy held from past experiences that were never fully expressed.
- **Energetic Pain** is a disruption in the body's natural flow of Qi, Prana, or life force.

When you release pain, you are essentially giving this blocked energy permission to move. This may show up as:

- A sudden **shift in pain** from one area to another.
- A wave of **heat, tingling, or vibration** in the body.
- An **emotional release** — tears, laughter, or sighs.
- A deep sense of **lightness or relief**, as though a weight has been lifted.

How to Support Energy Release with Quick Fix:

1. **Breathe Consciously:** Inhale into the point of tension; exhale as if pushing energy out of the body.
2. **Visualize Flow:** Imagine the pain dissolving into light or draining downward through the legs into the earth.
3. **Acknowledge the Message:** Silently thank your body for communicating. Recognition helps complete the release.

4. **Anchor the Shift:** After the sequence, rest your hands over your heart or navel to "seal in" the new balance.

Quick Fix Insight:
Releasing pain isn't just about removing discomfort — it's about restoring **flow.** When energy moves, the body heals, emotions balance, and the spirit feels free again.

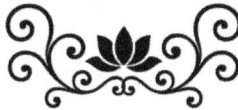

Building Your Daily Quick Fix Practice

MORNING & EVENING ROUTINES

One of the most powerful ways to transform Quick Fix from a simple pain-relief tool into a long-term wellness practice is to weave it into your daily rhythm. Just a few minutes in the morning and evening can reset your system, prevent tension from building, and keep your energy flowing smoothly.

Morning Routine – Starting Fresh

- **Why:** After a night's rest, your body may feel stiff or sluggish. Morning Quick Fix stimulates circulation, clears lymphatic congestion, and sets the tone for energy throughout the day.
- **How:**
    1. Begin with **light pounding on Point B (K24)** to wake up your chest and circulation.
    2. Run quickly through the full sequence (Points A–O), spending 10–15 seconds on each.

3. Finish with **deep breaths** and a moment of intention (e.g., *"Today I move with ease and energy."*)
- **Time:** 3–5 minutes

Evening Routine – Letting Go

- **Why:** Stress, tension, and emotional build-up from the day tend to lodge in the muscles by evening. A nighttime Quick Fix helps release this, preparing you for deeper, more restorative sleep.
- **How:**
  1. Begin at **Point B (K24)** with gentle rubbing instead of pounding to calm the system.
  2. Focus more time on **Points E (Heart), M (Lung), and H (Kidney)** — these are often overloaded by daily stress.
  3. Finish with **Point O (shoulder pinch)** to release the lower back and let the whole body relax.
  4. Take three slow, grounding breaths, exhaling the day's tension.
- **Time:** 5–7 minutes

Quick Fix Insight:
Think of your **morning Quick Fix** as *charging your battery* and your **evening Quick Fix** as *clearing the clutter*. Together, they keep your system balanced and resilient.

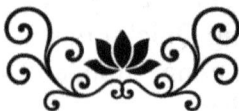

ON-THE-GO RELIEF

Pain doesn't wait for the perfect time or place. One of the strengths of the Quick Fix method is that you can use it anywhere — in your car, at work, or even in a bathroom when you need a private moment. With nothing more than your hands and a few minutes, you can interrupt pain before it takes over.

In the Car (Parked or at a Stoplight)

- Use **Point B (K24)** — light pounding or rubbing just under the collarbone helps you reset quickly if stress or tension builds while driving.
- Rub **Point N (outer thighs)** to ease hip or back stiffness from long drives.
- Gently pinch **Point O (shoulders)** at a red light to release lower back pressure.
  (Safety note: never attempt the sequence while the vehicle is in motion.)

At Work or in Public

- Step into a bathroom stall or a quiet hallway.
- Rub **Point H (Kidney, near the navel)** if you feel drained or anxious.
- Stimulate **Point E (Heart)** with firm circles if stress or emotions are overwhelming.
- If you have just 60 seconds, spend it on **Point B (K24)** — it's the fastest reset point.

Any Bathroom, Any Time

- I often tell clients, *"Your bathroom break can be your healing break."*
- Take one minute to rub **Point B (K24)** and then trace through a couple of chest points (A, E, M).
- End with three slow breaths while washing your hands — a discreet way to combine routine with relief.

Quick Fix Insight:
You don't need a mat, clinic, or quiet room to find relief. Quick

Fix works because it meets you where you are — whether that's in your car, at your desk, or in the middle of a busy day.

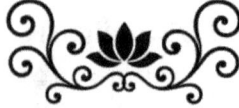

LONG-TERM BENEFITS

The Quick Fix method may provide immediate relief in minutes, but its real power is in the long-term results that come from consistent practice. Just as the body learns negative patterns of tension and pain, it can also **learn new patterns of balance, relaxation, and resilience.**

Physical Benefits

- **Fewer flare-ups:** Regular stimulation of neuro-lymphatic points helps keep muscles relaxed, reducing the risk of pain returning.
- **Improved posture and alignment:** By releasing tight muscles and balancing their opposites, your body holds adjustments more effectively.
- **Better circulation and lymphatic flow:** Supporting detoxification and oxygenation enhances overall vitality.
- **Stronger immunity:** Because many points are tied to immune and organ function, regular practice boosts resilience.

Emotional & Mental Benefits

- **Stress recovery:** With daily use, your nervous system becomes less reactive to triggers, making it easier to stay calm.
- **Emotional release:** Stored tension and unprocessed feelings find a pathway out, creating a sense of lightness and clarity.

- **Improved focus:** By calming background stress, the mind has more space for creativity, problem-solving, and presence.

Energetic & Spiritual Benefits

- **Balanced flow of Qi (life energy):** Restoring circulation through meridians creates harmony across body, mind, and spirit.
- **Deeper self-awareness:** Regular practice strengthens your connection to your body's signals.
- **Empowerment:** You no longer feel helpless against pain — you have tools in your own hands to respond and rebalance.

Quick Fix Insight:
The more often you practice Quick Fix, the less you'll need it for emergencies. Instead of being a "rescue technique," it becomes a lifestyle of balance — keeping pain at bay, energy flowing, and your body's wisdom alive at your fingertips.

Conclusion

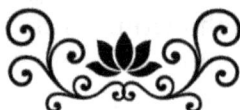

FROM QUICK FIX TO LASTING CHANGE

The Quick Fix was designed to bring you relief in moments —
and it does. But the real power of this method isn't just in the
immediate results; it's in what happens when you make it part
of your daily life.

Pain, whether physical, emotional, or energetic, is often the
body's way of signaling imbalance. The Quick Fix sequence
calms those signals, resets the nervous system, and restores
energy flow. When practiced regularly, it teaches your body a
new pattern: **relaxed muscles, balanced energy, and steady
resilience.**

Over time, this creates lasting change:

- **Muscles learn new habits.** Instead of pulling bones
  back out of alignment, they hold balance and ease.
- **Stress response resets.** The body becomes less reactive
  to daily triggers, and you bounce back faster.
- **Energy flows freely.** Lymphatic drainage improves,
  breathing deepens, and fatigue gives way to vitality.
- **Pain loses its grip.** Instead of being ruled by flare-ups,
  you gain the ability to manage discomfort and shorten
  recovery time.

The beauty of the Quick Fix is that it grows with you. At first, it may feel like a tool you reach for only when you hurt. But as you continue, it becomes a simple ritual woven into your day — in the morning, before bed, or whenever you need a reset.

Quick Fix Insight:
What begins as a quick remedy for pain often becomes a **daily practice for balance**. Over time, you'll discover that the Quick Fix isn't just about removing pain — it's about creating a body that feels lighter, a mind that feels calmer, and a life that feels more in flow.

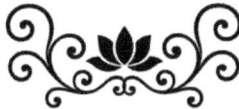

YOUR BODY'S WISDOM AT YOUR FINGERTIPS

Your body has always known how to heal. Every ache, every twinge, every knot of tension is its way of speaking to you — not as an enemy, but as a guide. Pain is not just a problem to be silenced; it is information, pointing toward imbalance and inviting you back into harmony.

The Quick Fix sequence gives you a simple way to listen and respond. With nothing more than your hands, your breath, and a few minutes of focus, you can unlock the body's natural wisdom. Each point you touch is more than a muscle or reflex — it is a doorway into balance, clarity, and vitality.

When you learn to trust these signals, you begin to understand that your body is not broken; it is brilliant. It holds deep intelligence in its tissues, rhythms, and energy flow. All it needs is your attention and care.

The power is — quite literally — **at your fingertips.**

Use it daily. Use it when pain flares up. Use it when you need calm, clarity, or strength. Over time, you will not only relieve pain but also cultivate a deeper connection to yourself — body, mind, and spirit working together.

Final Insight:
Healing doesn't always come from outside. Sometimes, the most profound medicine is already within you, waiting for your touch to awaken it.

Appendices

QUICK FIX PAIN RELIEF ACUPRESSURE CHART

Video Link

https://youtu.be/dQGnHNaW3_w

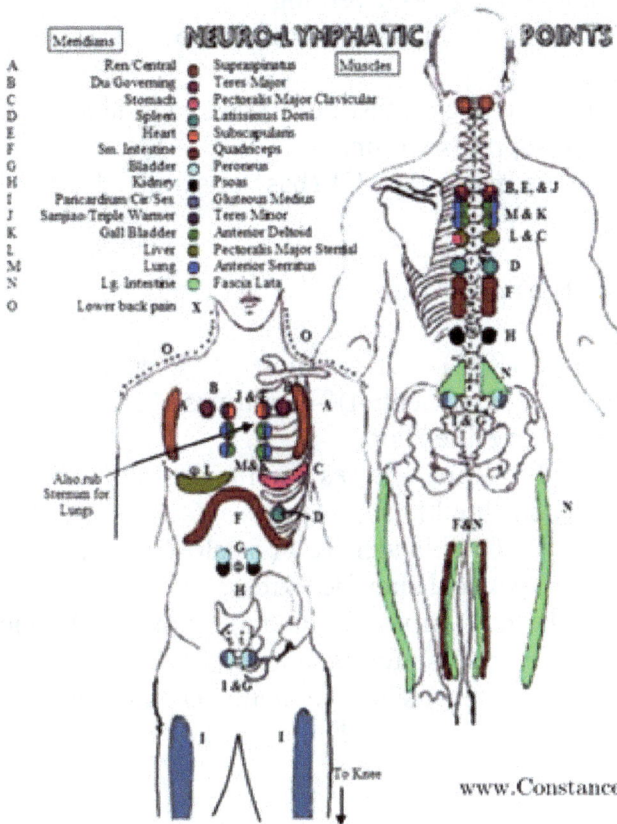

NEURO-LYMPHATIC POINTS

Meridians		Muscles	
A	Ren/Central	Supraspinatus	
B	Du Governing	Teres Major	
C	Stomach	Pectoralis Major Clavicular	
D	Spleen	Latissimus Dorsi	
E	Heart	Subscapularis	
F	Sm. Intestine	Quadriceps	
G	Bladder	Peroneus	
H	Kidney	Psoas	
I	Paricardium Cir/Sex	Gluteous Medius	
J	Sanjiao/Triple Warmer	Teres Minor	
K	Gall Bladder	Anterior Deltoid	
L	Liver	Pectoralis Major Sternal	
M	Lung	Anterior Serratus	
N	Lg. Intestine	Fascia Lata	
O	Lower back pain X		

B, E, & J
M & K
L & C
D
F
H
N

Also rub Sternum for Lungs

To Knee

F & N

www.ConstanceSantego.ca

QUICK REFERENCE SEQUENCES

These mini-routines pull from the full Quick Fix sequence and highlight the points most effective for specific issues. Use them when you're short on time or want to target a particular problem.

Headaches & Migraines

- **Start:** Point B (K24) – Governing reset, opens the chest.
- **Then:** Point K (Gallbladder) – Relieves neck/temple tension.
- **Then:** Point N (Large Intestine) – Clears fascia tension in hips/legs, supports elimination.
- **Finish:** Gentle massage at C1 (base of skull) – Releases suboccipital tension.

Neck & Shoulder Tension

- **Start:** Point B (K24) – Opens chest, resets energy.
- **Then:** Point A (Ren/Central) – Improves posture, releases front chest tension.
- **Then:** Point E (Heart) – Eases emotional strain and forward pull on shoulders.
- **Then:** Point K (Gallbladder) & J (Triple Warmer) – Relieve side-neck and shoulder stress.
- **Opposites:** Point I (Hips & buttocks) + Point G (Pelvic reflex) – Reflex release for shoulders.
- **Optional:** C1 (base of skull) for added neck relief.

Back Pain

- **Start:** Point H (Kidney) – Releases deep psoas/lumbar tension.
- **Then:** Point N (Large Intestine) – Stabilizes hips/IT band.
- **Then:** Point G (Bladder) – Supports sacrum and pelvis.

- **Finish:** Point O (Shoulder pinch) – Reflex release for lower back.
- **Optional:** Point A (Ren) + B (Du) for posture reset.

Stress & Anxiety

- **Start:** Point B (K24) – Nervous system reset.
- **Then:** Point E (Heart) – Emotional calming.
- **Then:** Point M (Pericardium) – Releases chest tightness, protects heart.
- **Then:** Point J (Triple Warmer) – Balances fight-or-flight response.
- **Finish:** Point A (Ren/Central) – Grounding and centering.

Fatigue & Low Energy

- **Start:** Point B (K24) – Light pounding to spark circulation.
- **Then:** Point H (Kidney) – Boosts core energy reserves.
- **Then:** Point M (Lung) – Deepens breath, increases oxygen.
- **Then:** Point D (Spleen) – Supports digestion and energy production.
- **Optional:** Point N (Large Intestine) to move stagnation.

Quick Fix Insight:
Each mini-sequence takes just 1–4 minutes. Use them as "first aid" for common issues, or combine them into your daily full-body Quick Fix practice.

QUICK FIX JOURNAL PAGES

Use these blank pages to record your experiences with the Quick Fix method. Writing down your pain levels, feelings, and results helps you see patterns and celebrate progress over time.

Daily Quick Fix Journal

Date: _____

Pain Location(s):

_____

Pain Level Before (1–10): _____

Points Focused On (circle or list):
A B C D E F G H I J K L M N O

Techniques Used:
☐ Rubbing
☐ Circular massage
☐ Light pounding (Point B)
☐ Shoulder pinch (Point O)
☐ Other: _____

Pain Level After (1–10): _____

Changes Noticed:
☐ Pain reduced
☐ Pain moved/shifted
☐ More relaxed
☐ Breathing deeper
☐ Emotional release
☐ Energy improved

Notes / Reflections:

_____

_____

_____

_____

Weekly Reflection Page

Week of: _____

- What pain or tension came up most often this week?

  _____

- Which Quick Fix points gave the best results?

  _____

- What changes did you notice in your body or mood over the week?

  _____

- Intention for next week:

  _____

Quick Fix Insight:
Journaling your progress helps you build awareness of your body's patterns. Many people discover that pain isn't random — it often reflects posture, stress, or emotional triggers. Tracking it makes it easier to break the cycle.

Bibliography

Much of this information was created and copyrighted when I owned the Canadian Institute of Natural Health and Healing Accredited College

Resources & Recommended Reading

These books and references have shaped the development of the Quick Fix method and can help you deepen your understanding of acupressure, kinesiology, energy medicine, and holistic self-care.

Foundational Texts

- Palmer, D.D. *The Science, Art and Philosophy of Chiropractic* (1895).
- Bennett, Terrence. *Neurovascular Reflex Therapy* (1930s clinical papers).
- De Jarnette, M.B. *Sacro-Occipital Technique Manuals* (1930s–1960s).
- Goodheart, George. *Applied Kinesiology: Research Manuals* (1960s).
- Thie, John. *Touch for Health: A Practical Guide to Natural Health with Acupressure Touch* (1973).

Acupressure & Energy Healing

- Gach, Michael Reed. *Acupressure's Potent Points: A Guide to Self-Care for Common Ailments.*
- Montakab, Mehrdad. *Acupuncture Point and Channel Energetics.*

- Motoyama, Hiroshi. *Theories of the Chakras: Bridge to Higher Consciousness.*
- Sancier, Kenneth. *Scientific Basis of Qigong and Acupressure.*

Kinesiology & Reflex Work

- Chapman, Frank. *Neurolymphatic Reflexes: Their Diagnostic and Therapeutic Value.*
- Diamond, John. *Life Energy: Using the Meridians to Unlock the Hidden Power of Your Emotions.*
- Kendall, Florence & Kendall, Henry. *Muscles: Testing and Function.*
- Walther, David. *Applied Kinesiology: Synopsis.*

Holistic & Self-Healing Practices

- Pert, Candace. *Molecules of Emotion: The Science Behind Mind-Body Medicine.*
- Chopra, Deepak. *Quantum Healing: Exploring the Frontiers of Mind/Body Medicine.*
- Nibley, Hugh. *Energy Medicine: The Scientific Basis.*
- Sills, Franklyn. *Foundations in Craniosacral Biodynamics.*

Additional Resources

- National Center for Complementary and Integrative Health (NCCIH) – https://nccih.nih.gov
- International Kinesiology College – https://www.ikc-info.org
- Touch for Health Kinesiology Association – https://www.touchforhealth.us

Note to Reader:

This list is not exhaustive, but it includes the pioneers and thinkers whose contributions paved the way for the Quick Fix method. Exploring these resources will deepen your appreciation of the body's innate intelligence and the many traditions that honor its ability to heal.

Message From The Author

When I first began this journey into natural health, I wasn't looking to write a book or create a method. I was simply searching for relief — for myself, for my family, and later for the clients who came to me in pain.

Like many of you, I learned firsthand that pain can be exhausting. It takes more than just a physical toll; it affects your mood, your confidence, and your ability to show up in life the way you want to. For years, I struggled with back pain that kept me from living fully. Chiropractic care would help, but the relief often didn't last. It wasn't until I discovered the power of neuro-lymphatic reflex points and began blending them with my background in energy medicine that something shifted. For the first time, I had a way to influence not just the spine or the muscles, but the *whole system* — body, mind, and energy together.

The Quick Fix method grew from those early discoveries. Over the years, I refined it in my clinic, teaching clients how to use it for themselves. What I noticed again and again was that when people were given tools they could use at home, they became more confident in their healing. Pain no longer ruled them — they had a way to respond, to shift it, and often to release it entirely.

This book is my way of passing that gift to you. It's not meant to replace your doctor, chiropractor, or therapist — they play an essential role. But it *is* meant to empower you with a simple, reliable way to listen to your body and take part in your own healing.

If there's one message I hope you carry with you, it's this: **your body is wise, and you have more power to help it heal than you may realize.** The Quick Fix is just one doorway into that wisdom. Use it when you're hurting, use it when you're tired, and use it as a daily ritual to stay in balance.

I am grateful that you've allowed me to share this with you. May this method bring you relief, resilience, and a renewed sense of trust in the intelligence of your body.

With warmth and encouragement,
Dr. Constance Santego

About the Author

Dr. Constance Santego is a bestselling author, educator, and natural medicine practitioner with over two decades of experience in holistic health and energy medicine.

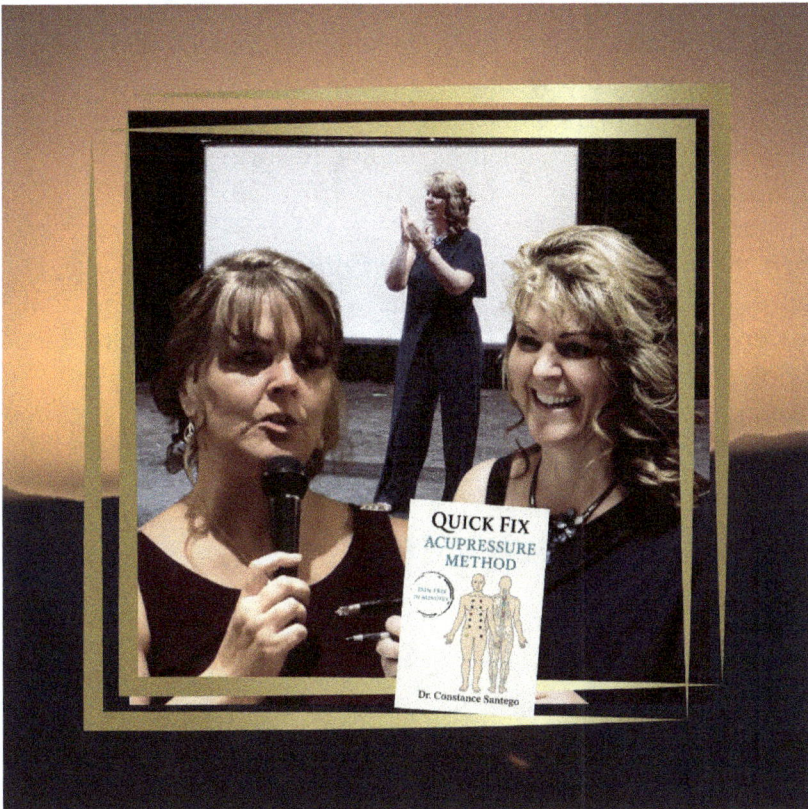

She holds both a Doctorate and Ph.D. in Natural Medicine and has trained thousands of students worldwide in modalities ranging from Reiki and acupressure to reflexology, aromatherapy, and intuitive development.

Dedicating her life to healing and teaching, Constance owned and operated an accredited college in natural health and esthetics in Canada, where she guided students through professional certifications and advanced healing studies. She has written more than forty books spanning nonfiction, practitioner manuals, and spiritual fiction, all rooted in her mission to empower others with tools for self-care, transformation, and resilience.

Her own journey with chronic back pain led her to discover the effectiveness of neuro-lymphatic reflex points — a breakthrough that became the foundation of the Quick Fix method. Blending the science of muscle memory with the wisdom of Eastern medicine, she developed this simple, accessible system for reducing pain and restoring balance in minutes.

When she's not teaching or writing, Constance enjoys life in beautiful British Columbia, Canada, where she finds inspiration in nature, community, and her family. Her passion remains helping others discover their innate ability to heal, grow, and live with greater vitality.

ALSO AVAILABLE

Secrets of a Healer, Magic of Muscle Testing

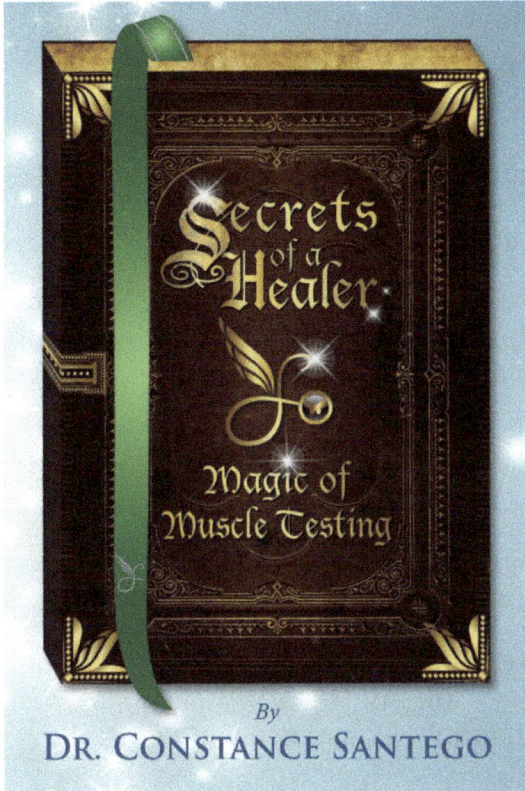

Magic of Muscle Testing is your guide to using **biofeedback techniques** to assess energy blockages, detect nutritional deficiencies, and restore balance naturally.

Start Healing Today!

Available in eBook & Softcover Format

eBook: https://constancesantego.ca/secrets-of-a-healer-magic-of-muscle-testing/

Softcover: ISBN: 9780978300531

Available at Barnes & Noble, Indigo/Chapters, Amazon

For additional information on

Constance Santego's

wide range of Motivational Products, Coaching Sessions,
Spiritual Retreats,
Live Events and Educational Programs

Go to

www.ConstanceSantego.ca

Follow on Instagram - Constance_Santego and
Facebook - constancesantegoo

Subscribe and receive Free Information and Meditations
on my
YouTube Channel - Constance Santego